Technology for Communication and Cognitive Treatment: The Clinician's Guide

A revolutionary approach to enhance treatment outcomes for people with speech, language, learning, and cognitive disabilities

By Joan L. Green, M.A., CCC, SLP

Innovative Speech Therapy ◆ Potomac, Maryland

Published and Distributed by:
Innovative Speech Therapy
7731 Tuckerman Lane #206
Potomac, MD 20854

ISBN 13: 978-0-9786942-5-8

For information about permission to reproduce selections from this guide, please contact Joan Green at www.ittsguides.com, write to: IST 7731 Tuckerman Lane, #206 Potomac, MD 20854, or call 1-800-IST-2550.

Trademark

Rather than put a trademark symbol with every occurrence of a trademarked name, we state that we are using the names to the benefit of the trademark owner, with no intention of infringement of the trademark.

Discounts

Products from Innovative Speech Therapy are available at bulk discounts for textbook course adoptions and for special promotions and fund-raising. For details, please contact Innovative Speech Therapy at www.ittsguides.com or call 1-800-IST-2550.

Warning: Disclaimer

The information provided is not to be viewed as professional consultation or services. This guide was designed to provide information about integrating the use of technology into communication and cognitive treatment. It is not the purpose of this guide to provide training for professionals, or prescribe evaluation or treatment protocols for clients. It was written to supplement the work of trained professionals in their efforts to help people with communication and cognitive challenges. Anyone who decides to integrate technology into education and rehabilitation must expect to invest time and effort into exploring and trying the suggested resources to learn which are best for particular individuals.

Every effort has been made to make this guide as complete and accurate as possible. However, there may be mistakes, both typographical and in content. It should be used as a general guide, not as the ultimate source of information. Many Web sites are provided for the reader to refer to for up-to-date information.

The author and Innovative Speech Therapy shall have neither liability nor responsibility to any person or entity with respect to any loss or damage caused, or alleged to have been caused, directly or indirectly, by the information contained in this guide. If you do not wish to be bound by the above, you may return this guide to the publisher for a full refund.

Books can be ordered online at www.ittsguides.com.

Technology for Communication and Cognitive Treatment:
The Clinician's Guide

A revolutionary approach to enhance treatment outcomes
for people with speech, language, learning,
and cognitive disabilities

A must-read for the following professionals:

- Academic development specialists
- Assistive technology specialists
- Educational consultants
- Learning disabilities teachers
- Neurologists
- Occupational therapists
- Physiatrists
- Professors
- Reading specialists
- Researchers
- Social workers
- Speech-language pathologists
- Technology coordinators
- Vendors
- Administrators
- Case managers
- Graduate students
- Media specialists
- Neuropsychologists
- Pediatricians
- Product developers
- Psychologists
- Recreational therapists
- School counselors
- Special educators
- Teachers
- Tutors

Table of Contents

Testimonials

Here's what professionals have written:

"I am deeply impressed with this work. It shows a great deal of knowledge about computers, but, more than that, it tells how to apply computers to your area of expertise. In my experience, this is something that is sorely needed, not just in your area of expertise, but in many other non-computer professions."

Mike Burks
Chairman, ICDRI (International Society for Disability Resources on the Internet)

"Thanks so much for a copy of the Technology Guide. It is incredible! I was amazed at the amount of information and detail included, and am hugely impressed that this has taken a *tremendous* amount of work and research."

Pat Latham Bach, Psy.D., RN

"WOW! This is going to be a very helpful tool! Joan, what an effort, and what a contribution. I am grateful and I applaud you!"

Darlene S. Williamson, M.A., CCC/SLP
Executive Director, Stroke Comeback Center

"Computer speech programs that exist today to help regain cognitive and communication skills are overwhelming for clinicians to learn about on their own. I absolutely endorse the use of this guide in graduate speech pathology programs. In addition, every clinical rehabilitation program should have these materials as a reference. It should be a required addition to the bookshelf of every professional involved in rehabilitation and special education.

Joan Green is to be applauded for having the vision, the energy, and the extensive knowledge base for compiling technological information into book format for clinicians to help their clients regain and return to optimum function. In my opinion, Joan is the leading expert in the country in helping people learn how to utilize computer applications to maximize their recovery."

Jill Arends, M.A., CCC-SLP
Comprehensive Speech Pathology Services, LLC

"Joan is uniquely qualified to apply and adapt software programs to meet the specific needs of her clients with communication and cognitive deficits. I have attended several of Joan's workshops and always found her presentations to be full of easily understood and highly useful information. I am sure that this guide will be of significant benefit to forward-thinking communication and education professionals."

Janet M. Gritz, M.A., CCC-SLP
Founder of Communication Matters

> "Your guide is wonderful. It is clear that you have put incredible energy into making it thorough and useful for a broad range of clinicians. I have recently added a cognitive rehabilitation component to my neuropsychology practice and am delighted to find information regarding so many resources in one place. I will definitely let others know about this timely, exceedingly pertinent resource. Most important, people in need of developing and restoring cognitive functions will benefit from your efforts! Thank you."
>
> Diane H. Engelman, Ph.D.

"I am thrilled that Joan Green is publishing her *Technology for Communication and Cognitive Treatment: The Clinician's Guide.* After being mentored by Joan on how to incorporate a variety of applicable training software, the Internet, screen readers, and other technology, I realized this opened a new door into how to approach therapy for my clients and their families. I believe that the suggestions by Joan Green will serve as an excellent resource for clinicians and as instructional material for graduate students at the university level who need to be aware of how to integrate technology into treatment approaches and life skills for their clients and their families."

Dede Matrangola, M.S., CCC-SLP
Instructor at Loyola College, Maryland

> "I am thoroughly impressed with Joan's level of expertise and professional excellence. I strongly support her unique treatment approach utilizing the most innovative technology tools available to maximize the language and cognitive potential of her clients. Her treatment regime is both motivating and reassuring as people with communication and cognitive challenges begin to experience progress they had not yet achieved with traditional treatment methods.
>
> Professionals in the fields of education and rehabilitation need to be trained in the uses of assistive technologies. Joan's guide for will help

ease the fear of those who are intimidated by 'technology' and in time will encourage more therapists to incorporate technology into their treatments. Joan gets results."

Elaine Schwartz, M.S. OTR/L
Creative Therapy Solutions

"Joan's suggestions for the design and equipment of our computer lab, as well as her recommendations and training of staff on the speech software was extremely valuable and helped us to get our program up and running effectively and efficiently. If we are training our therapists to offer long-term rehabilitation and they are not involving technology that has become as commonplace as the telephone, they are ignoring a life skill that can have a tremendous impact on the lifelong rehabilitation of an aphasic."

Karen Tucker, M.A.
Executive Director of Adler Aphasia Center

"Joan has written an invaluable resource for all professionals working with clients with communication and cognitive deficits. She is uniquely qualified to write this outstanding book, as her passion is to remove communication challenges through innovative technology applications. Joan is at the forefront of the paradigm shift of changing how we work with those who have cognitive and communication disorders. These are 21st century methods for a 21st century world!

Thank you, Joan for your thorough presentation of this material. I am a more knowledgeable consultant as a result of reading your book. This should be required reading in graduate programs throughout the country! There is no other comparable resource available."

Karen Janowski, M.S.Ed., OTL
EdTech Solutions, LLC

"The resource you are creating will be so beneficial to educators and clinicians who work with clients who have AT needs. The field of AT is so vast and ever-changing that it can be daunting; this comprehensive guide provides clinicians with detailed descriptions, rationales, and resources on this multifaceted topic in a clear, concise, and well-organized manner."

Patricia L. Mervine, M.A., CCC
Speaking of speech

"WOW — your guide is unique and thorough — congratulations!"

JoAnn Hoeppner, Ph.D.

"Let me congratulate you on such a huge undertaking! Wow!! From the chapters I read, it is a concise, well organized, and very useful collection of resources a clinician can use to implement technology into communication and cognitive therapy. I look forward to seeing this book and print. I will share it with my colleagues both in the clinical/rehab settings and the university settings. It is useful for students, new graduates, and seasoned clinicians. As you stated, our clients are always learning and so should we as clinicians."

Tami Brancamp, M.S./CCC-SLP

"I definitely think graduate students would benefit from this guide. The real world info is very valuable for a CFY."

Tara May, Graduate Student

"This looks just great! Thank you so much for your passion and taking the time, money, and effort to put this together. My hat is off to you."

Patty Banas, MACCC, SLP

"This will be a great reference tool for those therapists who wish to keep their therapy cutting edge and interesting for their patients."

Jon Lamere

"This impressive book provides a wealth of information. You would have to buy several other books to cover the content contained in this ONE book."

Mary Twentyman, Retired Elementary general and special education teacher

"Golden" Interactive Web Sites

treatment schedules are
ed, and it's time to think about
ucation Programs (IEPs) and
oplies. To get you in the mood
a smile or two by checking "IEPs
**nedsped.soe.umd.umich.edu/
n**). For more smiles, check out the
ctive Web sites with free materials
dapted to treatment.
are especially fun if you have
oard," which allows you to project
ktop in front of your classroom
ia.org/wiki/Interactive_whiteboard).
um (**www.gamequarium.com**) has
asures, including parts-of-speech
amequarium.com/partsofspeech.
er, different sound (**www.toonuniver-
asp?quizzes_key=18**); and Are You My
**.gamequarium.org/cgi-bin/search/
3431**).
s Literacy Zone (**www.woodlands-junior.
interactive/literacy/index.htm**) links to
ut words and spellings (including a link to
-like "Whomp"), grammar and punctuation,
t work, and online stories.
riteThink (**www.readwritethink.org**) offers
n of online student materials (**www.
ethink.org/student_mat/index.asp**) to
iteracy learning in the K-12 classroom. Three
vorites are "What's in the Bag?" (**www.
itethink.org/materials/in_the_bag/index.**
a game with clues provided for categorizing and
ulary; Word Family Sort (**www.readwritethink.
aterials/wordfamily**), an activity for recognizing
patterns and learning about onset and rhyme;
Picture Match! (**www.readwritethink.org/
erials/picturematch**), which offers practice identify-
beginning letters and short- and long-vowel sounds.

Online language arts games (**www.teachervision.
fen.com/reading-and-language-arts/games/5831.
html**) links to a large collection of materials for grades
Pre-K through 12.

Funbrain (**www.funbrain.com/kidscenter.html**)
has several games, including "Stay Afloat" (**www.
funbrain.com/hangman/index.html**) and MadLibs
featuring parts of speech (**www.funbrain.com/brain/
ReadingBrain/ReadingBrain.html**).

Internet4Classrooms (**www.internet4classrooms.
com/index.htm**) offers a listing of links, especially on
"language arts" (**www.internet4classrooms.com/
lang_gen.htm**); "language arts: elementary" (**www.
internet4classrooms.com/lang_elem.htm**); and
"language arts: elementary reading and writing" (**www.
internet4classrooms.com/lang_write_elem.htm**).

QUIA (**www.quia.com/shared**) templates can be
used to create a variety of activities, including concentration, matching, battleship, jeopardy, hangman, and
other fun formats. Enter "speech therapy" into the QUIA
search engine (**www.quia.com/shared**) to uncover
more than 450 interactive activities. Check out:

- Tracy Gefroh Boyd's articulation games (**www.quia.
  com/pages/havemorefun.html**), word/language
  games (**www.quia.com/pages/havefun.html**),
  and sequencing games (**www.quia.com/pages/
  sequencingfun.html**).

- Lonn Swanson's articulation activities (**www.quia.
  com/pages/speechersclass.html**); grammar
  games/activities (**www.quia.com/pages/grammar-
  crackers.html**); and vocabulary games (**www.quia.
  com/pages/worldowords.html**).

- Pamela Borda's links to literature games, idioms,
  antonyms, synonyms, conjunctions, word
  classes, and questions (**www.quia.com/pages/
  pbordashome.html**).

- Elaine Ramsay's articulation and phonological
  awareness games (**www.quia.com/pages/
  allpicturesfun.html**).

- Tina Dettbarn's activities (**www.quia.com/profiles/
  tdettbarn**).

- Jessica Braaten's activities (**www.quia.com/
  profiles/jbraaten**).

Language Guide (**www.languageguide.org/
english/**) teaches vocabulary, spelling, and pronunciation of several languages through pictures and audio.
It has more than 60 pages of categorized English
vocabulary from African animals to weather.

Scholastic (**www.scholastic.com**) offers many
great activities, including the categorization and
vocabulary-enriching activity "Nina Loves to Name
Things" at home, in the store, restaurant, firehouse,
farm, aquarium, supermarket, construction site, airport,
museum, garden, and zoo (**http://teacher.scholastic.
com/ACTIVITIES/bll/nina/index.htm**); I Spy (**www.
scholastic.com/ispy/play/healthyfun/index.asp**);
and the Magic School Bus (**www.scholastic.com/
magicschoolbus/games/sound**).

Grammar Blast (**www.eduplace.com/kids/
hme/k_5/quizzes/index.html**) has interactive quizzes
for grades 2–5.

Fun School's Language Games (**http://funschool.
kaboose.com/arcade/language/index.html**) has
games that build vocabulary and sequencing skills. ⬚

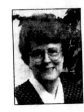

*Judith Maginnis Kuster, MS, CCC-
SLP, is a professor in the Department
of Speech, Hearing, and Rehabilitation
Services at Minnesota State University,
Mankato. Handouts from her 2009
ASHA Schools conference presenta-
tion are at **http://www.mnsu.edu/
comdis/2009schoolshandout.html**.*
*Contact her at judith.kuster@mnsu.edu. An archive of
Kuster's columns can be found at **www.mnsu.edu/
comdis/kuster4/leader.html**.*

by Judith Maginnis Kuster

School has started, probably establish... Individualized Ed... new equipment and su... for writing IEPs, enjoy... by Dr. Seuss" **(http://...belinda/iepsbydr.htm...** many "golden" intera... that can easily be a...

Interactive sites... access to a "whiteb... your computer des... **(http://en.wikiped...**

Game Aquari... a multitude of tre... games **(www.ga... html)**; same let... **sity.com/quiz....** Mother? **(www...linfo.cgi?id=...**

Woodland... **kent.sch.uk...** activities ab... the "Boggle... writing, tex...

ReadW... a collecti... **readwrit...** support... of my fa... **readw... html)**,... vocab... **org/...** word... and... **ma...** ing...

Acknowledgments

I am grateful to my family, friends, and colleagues for their continuous encouragement and support, even though this project took much longer than I ever imagined it would! I am continually helped and enriched by people who showed enormous faith and belief in my mission to spread the word about this use of technology to help others. Without them, I would not have been able to produce this guide.

I want to thank the following people:

- My supportive parents, Leah and Allan Lipman, for providing me with an enormous amount of help editing the chapters of this guide, offering insightful advice, and providing financial assistance to make this guide a reality

- My loving husband, Mark, for offering his encouragement and guidance along the way

- My children Hallie, Ilana, Elise, and Aaron for helping me explore the software and their enthusiasm and support — even though, at times, I wasn't able to offer them the attention they desired

- My brother, Bob Lipman, who guided me with creative suggestions and support and helped me create www.ittsguides.com

- My mother-in-law, Lilli Green, for helping to keep our house in order

- The many amazing clients and families I had the pleasure of helping who showed an enormous amount of dedication, diligence, and enthusiasm when using the technology to improve their lives. I learned a lot from them!

The many colleagues who helped review chapters, offer insightful suggestions, testimonials, and words of encouragement:

- Jill Arends, M.A., CCC-SLP

- Pat Latham Bach, Psy.D., RN

- Ruth Bluestone, M.A., CCC-SLP

- Tami Brancamp, M.S., CCC-SLP

- Karen Copeland, M.S., CCC-SLP

- Hindie Becker Dershowitz

- Jill Dosik, M.A., CCC-SLP

- Diane H. Engelman, Ph.D.

- Donna Finch, LCSW

- Nettie Fischer, ATP

- Janet Gritz, M.A., CCC-SLP

- JoAnn Hoeppner, Ph.D.

- Kevin Hsu

- Luann Jacobs, M.A., CCC-SLP, RMT

- Karen Janowski, M.S.Ed., OTL

- Judy Johnson, CCC/SLP, Ph.D.

- Scott Kashkin

- Jon Lamere

- Ginny Mahonny

- Dede Matrangola, M.S., CCC-SLP

- Tara May, Graduate Student

- Denise McCall, M.S., CCC-SLP

- Sharon Meldgin

- Patricia L. Mervine, M.A., CCC-SLP

- A. Simon Mielniczuk — Solutions Architect

- Sharon Newton, RN, Ph.D.

- Mark E. Nichols, M.Ed.

- Carol O'Day, Ph.D., CCC-SLP

- Lee Ohringer

- Thomas W. Powell, Ph.D.

- Barbara Sonies, Ph.D., CCC-SLP, BRS-S

- Barbara Thomas, M.A., CCC-SLP

- Mary Twentyman, Special Ed Teacher

- Candace Vickers, M.S., CCC-SLP

- Darlene Williamson, M.A., CCC-SLP

The many friends and professionals who helped guide me with the publishing process:

- Ann Litt, M.S., RD, LD
- Jill Mason, Editor
- Kathleen O'Connor, Editor
- RJ Communications
- Larry and Lisa London
- George Pasteur, PT

The many producers and sellers of products reviewed for inclusion in this guide and their often-generous donations.

Those who came to my rescue with computer questions:

- Susan Baer, Founder of Advanced Computer Learning
- Scott Miller, Founder of Giganet
- David Orenstein, M.L.S., M.S.
- Nerd Boy! Computers
- Dan Papetti, Interactive Employment Training
- Robert E. Simanski, Business Pro Services

About the Author

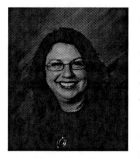 Joan Green, the founder of Innovative Speech Therapy, is passionate in her efforts to spread the knowledge of her exciting approach for helping people improve communication and cognition. Her expertise, developed over the past 20 years, involves integrating technology and other resources into treatment to help clients, patients, and students realize their potential with practical, efficient, and affordable solutions. Her mission is to empower people with disabilities to use the powerful tools of technology to improve their lives. Joan is concerned about people becoming discharged too soon from therapy due to the trend toward fewer reimbursable speech sessions.

Joan has spoken extensively to professionals, as well as clients and caregivers, at the local, state, and national levels to promote the integration of computers and technology into treatment. She leads professional workshops and speaks at a wide variety of seminars. Joan trains professionals and graduate students to incorporate technology into sessions. She consults with aphasia centers, regular and special education schools, assistive living facilities, hospitals, and rehabilitation centers, and senior centers to facilitate the coordination of computer based programs for people with communication and cognitive challenges. Joan attends many conferences and continues to very actively research potential therapy resources, products, and therapy techniques.

She is always looking out for new innovative ways to help her clients. Joan is the founder of two short-term technology oriented intensive programs in Potomac, Maryland.

TWIST for Adults is a customized intensive weeklong, speech therapy program. It was developed for stroke and head injury survivors, people who have degenerative neurological diseases, and adults with learning disabilities and other communication and cognitive challenges.

TWIST for Parents is a short-term intensive technology oriented training and coaching program for parents of children with language and learning challenges.

In additional to writing this book to help professionals learn to use the tools of technology to enhance treatment, she offers several training and consulting options to help people who work in the fields of education, rehabilitation and wellness jump-start their practice and speed up the learning curve.

- Workshops and seminars
- Consultation and coaching
- Online training

Joan plans to write several more books and e-books focused on helping people with aphasia, learning disabilities, developmental delays and other communication and cognitive challenges.

Joan received her undergraduate and graduate level education and training at Northwestern University. She grew up in Buffalo, NY, and lives in Potomac, MD with her husband Mark, their four children, and Honey — their yellow lab.

Introduction:
Suggestions for Using This Guide To Meet Your Immediate Objectives

You've been thinking about learning to use technology in your daily routines. Perhaps you want to introduce graduate students to the benefits of technology, need to increase revenue for your school or rehabilitation program, or you are searching for ways to improve client satisfaction. You've probably heard that the use of specialized software and adaptive hardware along with more traditional treatment often improves outcomes and makes treatment more enjoyable. Family members may be asking you what can be done to improve therapy results or what they can do on their own to speed up progress.

Until now, perhaps it has just been your goal to use technology. We are often too busy or overwhelmed to make that goal a reality. Another possibility is that you were not aware of the many resources available to help you do your job better. Each day we are consumed by multiple demands and there is often little time to explore options and to take the initiative to learn more about how effectively to integrate technology into practical solutions to improve or compensate for deficits pertaining to talking, listening, reading, writing, thinking, and remembering. We strive for the same objective — to deliver the best treatment possible and enjoy the process. This guide will help you with this mission.

The terms used to describe who we are, what we do, and who we help change depending on our professions and work settings. You may be a speech-language pathologist working in a school setting, a learning disabilities specialist in an evaluation center, an occupational therapist working in a hospital, a neuropsychologist with your own practice, a recreation therapist in a day treatment program, a media specialist in a rehabilitation center or a teacher of English as a second language in a clinic. Although some of you are therapists and others are doctors and teachers, in this guide I refer to professionals providing help to others as "clinicians." People who are helped in medical settings are referred to as "patients," people in schools are typically referred to as "students," and people who are in private practices are referred to as "clients." In this guide, although the provision of services can take place in a multitude of settings, I typically refer to the people being helped as "clients." Our jargon describing what we do in different surroundings also differs. We may be involved in "teaching," "treatment," "training," "coaching," "consulting," "counseling," or "evaluating." I use a variety of these terms throughout this guide.

I have spoken to many large groups of professionals as well as consumers and have been told repeatedly that the methods I use in my practice are innovative. My training programs and lectures serve to motivate and encourage professionals to take the plunge and get started implementing technology into their programs. I hope that this guide will have the same effect for you and inspire you to initiate this learning process. Most clinician's realize that they would probably benefit from learning how to use technology to improve their service delivery and treatment outcomes. They often don't know where to begin, have become overwhelmed in their attempts to learn, or just don't have the time, money, or inclination to get started.

I wrote this guide to make this seemingly insurmountable task of learning more about the use of technology within reach. Clients deserve to be exposed to this information, strategies, and treatment methods. I have tried my best to organize and share what I have learned during the past 20 years into a format that will help others benefit from my experiences. I embarked on this project about three years ago and never imagined that it would take me so long to finish! I wanted this guide to be as complete as possible, so that it could be used as a resource to help a wide variety of professionals who work in many different settings with people who have many different communication and cognitive related issues.

As I researched the software, devices, and online resources, the enormity of this task became evident. Just when I thought I was done, I discovered more to include in this guide. I am sure that even with this effort to make this guide as comprehensive as possible, I have probably left out helpful resources. I will continue to explore Web sites, read the literature, and check out new products, as they are made available. I realize that new Web sites will be formed and prices may increase or decrease after publication. In order to keep this information current, I plan to create online products such as e-books which can be easily updated which will provide more detailed information on products discussed in this guide and highlight new resources and products that can help improve the lives of people with communication and cognitive deficits as they become available. E-books will be available at www.ittsguides.com.

I consulted with many professionals who are new to this world of technology, and was encouraged to start with a book that readers could hold while exploring Web sites and software. I also spoke with many neuropsychologists, assistive technology specialists, speech-language pathologists, occupational therapists, and special educators to learn more about their experiences with technology and asked them to review chapters of this guide in order to make it as helpful as possible to as many professionals as I could. I really want to expedite the process of moving our professions forward. This is the flagship product in a series I am producing and publishing called "Innovative Technology Treatment Solutions."

I have done my best to research, acquire, review, and use products with as many clients as possible in my practice. I have personally used the majority of the products listed in this guide and explored many online sites. However, there are products included in this guide that I have not used personally, but have reviewed online and are deemed worthwhile from other experienced professionals. I didn't want to omit helpful resources just because I have not used them.

With the help of this comprehensive guide, you can start to use or expand your use of technology to help others. It is only a matter of time until all clinicians will be expected to know much of this information. Whether you are a seasoned clinician with many years of experience, or a graduate student just starting out, the keys to success in using this guide are the same:

- Start gradually. Continue to do what you do best in your current practice and slowly add new technique incorporating the tools described in this guide.

- Focus on the sections within chapters first that will meet you immediate needs. This guide is not meant to be read cover to cover. It will be too overwhelming.

- Read Chapters 1, 2, and 3 prior to selecting the additional chapters that pertain to you. Chapter 2 presents information that I have perceived to be the most worthwhile according to the setting in which professionals work. My "top picks" are listed for each setting. Chapter 3 presents my "technology tips" for getting started organized by area of disability and deficit. I write brief scenarios to help readers envision how the described resources can be used to help.

Here are a few scenarios that describe how you may begin to read this guide:

- If you want to learn more about networking with other professionals in situations similar to yours, find an online support group for a family member, or research potential treatment options for a new client with a diagnosis with which you are not all that familiar you could start by reviewing Chapter18, "Online Support, Information, and Discussion Groups."

- If your goal is to seek guidance in applying for a grant to form a computer lab or have you just been given money to use for your clinic start by reviewing Chapter 2, "Treatment Settings," and read about my "top picks" for your workplace. Chapter 7, "Supportive Research," will point you in the direction of objective research data to support the claim that your clients will benefit from the software and hardware you select for purchase. Chapter 6, "Computer Setup Considerations," will help you figure out what you need to consider when setting up your lab.

- Perhaps you have a new client with severe verbal apraxia who benefits from drill and repetition while seeing up close-mouth movement. Chapter 8, "Treatment and Technology To Improve Verbal Expression," would be a great chapter to review first.

- If your budget is virtually nonexistent, but you really want to be able to show your clients and students what they can do online to reach their goals faster, start out by reviewing Chapter 16, "Games and Free Online Interactive Activities."

- Perhaps you want to make your sessions more engaging or find yourself spending too much time creating therapy materials and want to explore ways to produce customized materials more efficiently. If this describes your current situation, check out Chapter 15, "Multi-Media Programs and Generating Printed Treatment Materials."

This book assumes that you are skilled at evaluating your clients and providing traditional treatment. It also assumes that you have a basic knowledge of computer use such as: word processing, e-mail, Web site access and online searches and that you are open to new ideas to enhance your sessions. This guide will help you learn more about terms relating to technology, rehabilitation, and education in the glossary. It will also expose you to the many available resources so that you can learn where to go for help and where to search for information that is more detailed.

Once you select software, adaptive hardware or suggested online sites that are potentially helpful for your setting — spend some time exploring the Web sites that are given for the products discussed. Many businesses offer free demo CDs, a trial period for online subscriptions, or online tutorials. Another helpful feature offered by some vendors is the ability to join a listserv, participate in chat sessions, receive free e-newsletters, or access a bulletin board that will connect you to other users of the product. Promotions and discounts for many products are available by entering codes that may be found on my Web site at www.ittsguides.com.

I wrote this book to help improve the quality of life for people who have communication and cognitive deficits. We are in this together. My goal is to help you learn more about the many resources and potential solutions that will improve your treatment. I offer a variety of professional training and coaching programs, as well as intensive technology based treatment programs for clients and parents that are described on my treatment- and training-oriented Web site at www.innovativespeech.com. If you have general questions or comments, please feel free to contact me at Joan@innovativespeech.com.

I hope that you find that this guide is worthwhile. Please feel free to contact me if you have suggestions about how to improve this guide or know of additional resources that ought to be included with future revisions.

Chapter 1:
Why Use Technology?

A New Treatment Paradigm

Technology has slowly crept into our professional and personal lives. Assistive technology (AT) has become an integral part of this evolution and is gaining increased acceptance in the delivery of rehabilitation and special education services. We are in the midst of a paradigm shift involving our approach to helping others to improve their communication and cognition. This change is a process, not a one-time event. It is a new vision that our professions must embrace in order to provide the highest level of care possible. Educational and health-care systems are struggling to balance the delivery of quality services with increasing costs. With the use of the strategies and technologies demonstrated in this guide, clinicians become empowered to revolutionize treatment delivery to people of all ages with a wide range of communication and cognitive challenges.

The use of computers in therapy first appeared in the late '70s with the advent of microcomputers. Word processors gradually replaced typewriters. The primary function of computer use with clients was for word processing. In the '80s, computer use in therapy progressed to the use of drill-and-practice exercises that closely resembled workbook activities, but provided instant feedback. This feedback facilitated the learning process. The '90s ushered in easier access to the Internet and more sophisticated software programs with voice output, the ability to customize options in programs for clients, and more interesting and interactive software. Treatment started to incorporate the use of e-mail and Web sites for reading practice, research, and promotion of self-advocacy.

We are now in the midst of a second technology transformation that offers us even greater opportunities to help our clients. This new technology enables us to advance even further in helping people of all ages who have communication and cognitive challenges. We have reached a pivotal point and need to change our mind-set from using only traditional treatment to prioritizing the establishment of sustained efforts to integrate technology into our services.

Help for the Disabled

People challenged by disabilities can benefit from technology in many aspects of their lives. Computers and other devices, when selected and used with the help of a skilled clinician, can help improve communication and cognitive skills related to education, employment, recreation, and social and medical needs. AT can help individuals increase independence, build self-confidence and self-esteem, and improve quality of life.

Better, more affordable technology holds great promise for individuals with disabilities. Some professionals have welcomed this development of new resources to help others with open arms, some have avoided, resisted, or ignored these helpful tools, and others are unaware that new and exciting treatment opportunities exist. Children and adults with a broad range of difficulties resulting from strokes, head injuries, degenerative diseases, developmental delays and disorders and learning differences can independently handle a wider range of activities with the help of software and devices to read, write, organize, remember, learn, communicate, and search for information.

Disabilities Hinder an Individual's Ability To Benefit From Mainstream Computer Use

Communication and cognitive deficits create obstacles to computer use. As technology becomes even more important to mainstream society, people who do not have ready access to a computer or the Internet and are not exposed to support from skilled professionals will be at an increasing disadvantage.

It may be difficult for individuals with communication and cognitive challenges to

- provide computer input with movement of a mouse or typing on the keyboard,
- read and interpret information on the monitor,
- sequence and analyze procedures needed to use software applications,
- use e-mail to obtain information and interact socially, and/or
- surf the Web.

The Need for Professionals To Learn To Use Technology

Professionals who want to deliver top-quality therapy need to learn to integrate technology into treatment. A significant number of schools, rehabilitation centers, and private practices have already purchased computers, but many clinicians do not know how to use the technology as an effective therapy tool. Early efforts toward the use of computers in therapy concentrated on setting up the infrastructure — the hardware, software, and networking — that has become more affordable. As further hardware developments occur with wireless labs, faster computer processors, increased storage capacity, and improved Web applications, an emphasis needs to be placed on training clinicians to use creatively these tools to promote improved outcomes.

This professionally oriented guide is designed for clinicians who strive to be current and to maximize the effectiveness of their work. It has been extensively peer-reviewed by a wide variety of specialists who work in many different settings. This new therapy approach, with the strategies and tools presented in the following chapters, can make a tremendous difference and act as a catalyst for progress.

Appropriately, selected materials can

- save time;
- motivate clients;
- make the clinician's work easier;
- support unique learning styles, abilities, and backgrounds;
- facilitate positive outcomes;
- streamline data collection; and
- provide opportunities to objectively document change over time.

Many Different Types of Clients Can Benefit From Computer Use in Therapy

Many new, powerful devices and software programs have been developed to help people confronted with a wide variety of challenges. People who are appropriate candidates for learning support from computers may have experienced or still have the following:

- A brain insult such as a stroke, a closed-head injury, a tumor, or an aneurysm

- A progressive degenerative disease such as Parkinson's, amyotrophic lateral sclerosis (ALS), or multiple sclerosis (MS)

- A cognitive decline

- Mild cognitive impairment

- Poor performance in school

- Work-related challenges

- Unintelligible speech

- Dysfluent speech

- Difficulty learning English as a second language

- A developmental delay or disorder

- Developmental apraxia of speech

- Intellectual impairment

- Autism

- A learning disability

- A voice disorder

- Hearing impairment

- Low vision

As computers continue to become more powerful, less expensive, and more portable, they are increasingly helpful in improving speech, language, new learning, reasoning, and memory. By creating opportunities as well as removing performance barriers, technology can help us explore new frontiers in meeting our clients' needs.

There Is a Lack of Experienced Clinicians Who Use Technology

Finding qualified help is often a difficult process for many clients. The training of clinicians to use these new tools is a time-consuming endeavor with many barriers. Clinicians who desire to develop an expertise in this area are often discouraged by a lack of time, guidance, or money to learn about and implement available treatment resources. Consequently, many clients are not exposed to the numerous benefits of computer use in the learning process.

There are many reasons for this dearth of available help:

- There is a global shortage of qualified and experienced communication and cognitive specialists.

- Reimbursement for treatment is increasingly hard to come by.

- Limited funds have drastically reduced the number of therapy sessions covered by insurance.

- Students in schools are generally seen by specialists for individual therapy only if they have very significant speech and language deficits that affect academic performance.

- Many communication disorders and special education programs do not provide sufficient training on the use of technology in the treatment process.

- There are not enough readily available continuing education opportunities to learn about this treatment approach.

- It is very costly and time consuming to explore software independently on the market to find which would be best for the situation, order it, try it and learn it, and then figure out how to use it to reach therapy goals.

Clinical Judgment and Experience Is Critical for Success

If clinicians could use a "cookie cutter approach" for integrating technology into treatment, the solution to this shortage would be much easier. However, developing an appropriate technology-based program for clients is a challenging process. No single hardware or software product addresses each person's unique communication and cognitive profile and specific needs. A variety of resources is most often needed. Products should be used in different ways with different clients. Clinical judgment is a critical component of individual assessment and effective program implementation. Many of the resources discussed are not produced for clients with disabilities and special needs. These clients need a creative clinician to establish the most helpful way to use the software or device to help reach therapy goals.

Family Advocacy Pushes Professionals To Learn About Technology

People who seek the services of clinicians who work in the fields of education and rehabilitation are very appreciative when exposed to software, devices, resources, and strategies that may help them or their loved ones reach their greatest potential. When information about such things is withheld, clients who later learn about these resources may become frustrated that they had not been made aware of products available for their empowerment.

Often the family members of people with disabilities take the initiative to learn more about treatment options. They expect their clinicians to use state-of-the-art treatment approaches. These people confront the devastating impact every day that the loss imposes on most aspects of daily life and are very motivated to seek alternative solutions to maximize progress and quality of life.

This Guide Is a Needed Resource for Clinicians

This guide streamlines the learning process and makes it more affordable for professionals to offer technology as a tool in their sessions. Computer-based tools and other resources have strengths and weaknesses. None can replace a clinician in the therapy process, but therapists and clients who understand what these new tools can do in solution-focused therapy to supplement other techniques can achieve excellent results. This Guide was created to help professionals overcome the many obstacles and consider the use of technology more effectively, efficiently, and at far less expense.

New devices with improved features and expanded capabilities continue to be developed. As we look toward the evolution of this rapidly improving technology and toward our profession embracing it, consumers will expect clinicians to be well versed in these techniques. We will also be expected to demonstrate how our therapeutic approaches can help facilitate actual functional changes.

Incorporating computers and technology into rehabilitation and education is well worth the effort, time, motivation, and dedication it requires. This guide highlights software, hardware, and other resources that are versatile and therapeutically beneficial. The items mentioned are not an exhaustive list of instructional tools and strategies, but rather a representative sampling of products available on the market and some suggestions about how to use them.

Benefits of Computer Use

Integrating computers into therapy sessions provides many benefits:

It's Interesting, Practical, and Fun

- The use of software, the Internet, and other devices is helpful because it maintains interest and avoids repetition and boredom. Computer use adds a different dimension to treatment for both the therapist and the client.

- Sessions can readily engage a client when the focus is on a particular interest, hobby, or current event.

- A creative therapist can work toward a wide variety of targeted goals, while the content relates to the client's area of appeal.

- Reading and writing practice can have real-life value when used with e-mail to friends and family.

- Practice using products that offer support for memory and organization can offer immediate, daily guidance for real life situations.

- Practice can take the form of enjoyable games.

It Offers the Ability To Control Tasks

Technology provides feature flexibility and customizability at a level previously impossible. Some software provides the ability to fine-tune tasks to allow for incremental changes.

It is now possible with some programs to customize the user interface and modify the feature set for each individual.

When using tasks that involve following directions, the clinician can select whether there is auditory or written stimuli, or both. The number of critical elements provided can be selected. The number of foils and the type of feedback and criteria for moving to a more difficult level can be controlled.

If the goal is to improve speech intelligibility, the selection of the target sound, its position within the word, the use of up-close videos of mouth movement, and the type of feedback can be selected. In addition, the ability to record the client's utterance, provide feedback on the accuracy of the speech, and use of sentence completion cues can be very effective.

It Gives Independent, Nonjudgmental, Immediate Feedback

Clients who may be defensive when a therapist or family member indicates that they provided an incorrect response may respond better when a computer provides feedback. It is often perceived as less personally threatening or controversial. Clients can benefit from the routine of the software and the predictable nature of the computer. When working with family members, this is not always the case. It is also possible to customize the type of feedback (auditory, visual or both) provided that will encourage continued participation.

Computers Promote Effective Independent Practice

Practice between sessions and frequent repetition is important for the carryover of new behaviors. Computers can promote this new learning by

- enabling people to practice exercises or complete tasks many times,
- providing immediate feedback,
- freeing clients of the dependence on others to practice, and
- making it easier for a "computer buddy" to assist with the assignment.

It Maximizes the Effectiveness of Limited Treatment Sessions

Sufficient reimbursement from insurance companies and other third-party payers is becoming increasingly difficult to obtain; consequently, the number of visits has been slashed. Clients need an effective way to practice between sessions to maximize their independent progress. This enables the therapist to be freed up to work on other tasks during therapy that the computer cannot replicate. Visits can be scheduled further apart once a client can improve more on his or her own in order to maximize their productivity.

It Provides Solutions To Improve Quality of Life Quickly

Several computer-based applications can quickly provide compensatory strategies to greatly improve a variety of abilities.

- Clients who have good auditory comprehension skills, but poor reading comprehension skills may learn to use a screen reader in just one or two sessions. The computer will read aloud what they select. They may then be able to enjoy an online newspaper, read e-mail from a friend, or read bills or recipes scanned into their computer.

- Clients who have difficulty with visual skills such as quick localization or eye tracking may benefit from text-to-speech software that highlights each word as it is read.

- Individuals who are unable to write, but who speak clearly and have good cognitive skills may benefit from voice-recognition software. It enables them to talk and have the computer type what they say.

- People who can write, but have difficulty thinking of words and organizing written narrative may benefit from graphic organizers to help brainstorm and write coherent messages and documents.

- Word prediction technology and online dictionaries are helpful for people who have difficulty thinking of words.

- Clients who have problems keeping track of daily activities may benefit from handheld electronic organizers.

- People who have difficulty communicating basic needs may benefit from devices with which they can select pictures or words and have the computer speak for them.

Increased Profitability

Once treatment incorporates technological advances, more rapid progress is often observed. This increased client satisfaction generates new business and the ability to charge more for services. Administrators, investors, grant providers, and practice owners will be pleased with the increased revenue that is created.

Help Is Available When There Is a Shortage of Professionals

Computer-savvy professionals are often strapped for time because their skills are in such high demand. Clients can travel to experienced clinicians, receive a comprehensive assessment and a comprehensive technology-based practice program, and then work on their own to achieve their goals. After practicing on their own or with the help of another person, they can return to the clinician as needed for independent practice program changes and updates.

Technology Offers Control for Family

Technology provides a way for clients to continue therapy independently at home. Family members who encourage this type of therapeutic carryover often feel empowered. Many people may feel too dependent on others if they believe their only option is to rely on the expertise of others. Many are not aware of the ways they can work at home to enhance the treatment.

Chapter 2:
Getting Started

This guide is structured to maximize the effectiveness of the time you devote to incorporating technology into treatment. It is organized so that you can find pertinent information quickly. Change...

From:	To:
"I don't have enough time."	"This resource saves me time!"
"I wouldn't even know where to start."	"I now know where to start."
"I'm not good with computers."	"Using computers is easier than I thought."
"It would cost too much money."	"I didn't realize how many free resources there are."
"I won't be able to do it."	"I can do this!"
"It won't help."	"Is it time to update my repertoire of tools?"
"There is too much to learn."	"My clients are learning new skills; so must I."
"My clients don't need it."	"My clients are consumers who are asking for it."
"It's too expensive."	"It's too expensive not to consider technology."

Many communication and cognitive specialists have thought of at least one of the above "change" statements when considering how technology could enhance their treatment. It is my hope that your experience in reading this guide and in learning about the many solutions available will be a painless and perhaps even enjoyable process. My intention is not to train professionals how to evaluate a client or how to provide speech, occupational, reading, writing, or other treatment. My goal is to encourage everyone involved in the rehabilitation and education process to work together using the best tools, resources, and treatment strategies available to help maximize the potential for people with communication and cognitive challenges. It is our responsibility as professionals to offer our clients the most updated and appropriate tools to maximize successful outcomes.

First Steps

Step 1: Facilitate your learning.

- Look at your surroundings, and make sure that they are conducive to learning. Most of us do best if we limit our distractions and focus on one thing at a time.

- Keep this guide near your computer, so that you can quickly access Web sites of interest as you prepare for sessions and initially read through these chapters.

- Be ready to highlight pertinent information to make it your own. I suggest that as you review the material, you place sticky notes on pages with the names of clients who might benefit from a particular resource or technique.

Step 2: Review this guide.

- Each reader will use the information provided in a different way. We all work in different settings, possess unique therapy approaches, and help many different types of clients who have diverse goals.

- Flip through the contents, and highlight the chapters that apply most to your current situation. Prioritize what you need to explore first, so that you can get up and running as fast as possible.

Step 3: Focus on your reasons for reading this guide.

- As a speech-language pathologist, occupational therapist, case manager, tutor, doctor, learning disabilities specialist, special educator, school or hospital administrator, university professor, researcher, product developer or graduate student, there are many reasons you might want to learn more about using technology as part of treatment. New information is most effectively learned when it is related to particular situations and when there are immediate opportunities in which to use it.

The following are possible reasons for reading this book:

- To help others improve their communication and cognitive abilities

- To help others compensate for deficits to improve their overall quality of life

- To make therapy sessions and independent practice assignments more interesting, effective, and enjoyable for clients

- To help others research conditions, medications, and treatments

- To make your job more interesting and fun

- To improve the outcomes of treatment sessions

- To learn about evidence-based, effective, state-of-the-art treatment approaches

- To research potential treatment solutions for clients

- To assist clients with returning to work

- To help students become more successful in school

- To help others explore leisure, educational, work, community re-entry, and social pursuits

- To develop helpful products

- To create lucrative and successful education and rehabilitation programs

- To learn more about potential treatment approaches in order to refer people to the most appropriate clinicians

- To identify barriers to success and determine solutions that promote independence

Step 4: Make a plan.

- Some of you may quickly fly through the contents and be eager to get started. You may be able to spend several hours each day reading this material and referring to the Web sites listed for potential treatment solutions.

- Others of you may be overwhelmed with current obligations and may have to take a slower approach, perhaps targeting two thirty-minute sessions a week. Make appointments with yourself to accomplish these tasks, and record them in your calendar.

Step 5: Locate appropriate resources for your particular needs.

- As mentioned in the Introduction, start out by looking at the section in Chapter 3 that focuses on your particular work setting. "Top picks" are listed for each setting. Chapter 4 lists suggestions for getting started with particular types of clients who are presented in 10 scenarios.

- Chapter 19 lists helpful organizations and listservs for your profession as well as for the diagnoses and disabilities with which you work. The Web sites listed provide a wealth of very valuable information. There is also quite a bit of helpful information on the sites listed which offer assistive technology training and information.

- Once you decide what you want to focus on to get started, go back, and read the chapters in this guide which focus on particular goal areas and types of resources that are available. There is a product index and a vendor index at the end of the book to help you quickly locate where particular resources are mentioned. Items are often discussed in more than one section of the book.

Therapy Focus and Customized Approach

Many professionals are reluctant to use technology in their practice and many administrators in graduate level training programs have been unwilling to introduce this material to their students. People who resist integrating technology into education and rehabilitation are usually under the false impression that when computers are used as an integral part of therapy, the clinician will seat the client at the computer and let the computer take the lead. The people who feel that it's inappropriate to use computers as a therapy might also erroneously believe that computer software enables clients to help themselves sufficiently — so much so that trained and certified professionals are no longer needed.

Software should not dictate the therapy. The needs of the person seeking help should influence the type of software selected. It's important to first carefully analyze the strengths and weaknesses of the individual's communicative and cognitive profile. Therapy goals need to be related to improving functional aspects of daily living, educational or vocational pursuits, or social and leisure activities.

Although computers are helpful in the therapy process, they do not replace specialized training with professionals. Users of the technology need to remain focused on the goals of therapy and work to achieve the desired outcomes. Once software is selected, it should be adapted and used to help the individual in the best way. People learn in different ways, and are helped by different strategies and types of assistance. Communication and cognitive professionals are trained to help people with communication and cognitive deficits, and computers are only a tool to further that help. One product can be used in many ways. Figuring out the way to use the technology is critical for success. Computers are used not only for remediation and rehabilitation but also to accommodate for deficits. Computers can remove the barriers to independence and success especially when used in the client's natural setting such as their home, school, or workplace.

Creating Flexible and Interesting Multimedia Practice Programs

After the strengths, weaknesses, and needs of the client have been comprehensively analyzed, it's necessary to obtain a clear picture of the client's daily life and what additional supports he or she has. It's also necessary to talk about where and when the technology will be used.

Clients or computer buddies, who are helping the client as needed, should be able to demonstrate during treatment sessions that they're able to appropriately practice exercises or software use prior to having them assigned as part of their practice program. The users also need to know what to change if the exercises become too easy or too hard, so that practice time remains productive. It's also important that the assignments are diverse enough to address therapy needs while providing enough variety to prevent boredom.

Computer Access

To initiate the use of computer technology in treatment, a reliable method of access to the computer should be established first. When a client needs an alternative access mode such as a foot switch, eye gaze, or other method, it may be necessary to refer the client to a major rehabilitation center or to another professional with the specialized expertise. Once the optimal method of computer access has been achieved, it is then possible to select and train the client to use the software that can help maximize rehabilitation outcomes.

Several products on the market and a few free online protocols were produced to help professionals assess where to start with computer access and software selection.

Title	Website	Price	PC	Mac	Online
The SETT Framework	http://sweb.uky.edu/~jszaba0/SETTintro.html	Free	x	x	Download
WATI	www.wati.org	Free	x	x	Download
COMPASS	www.kpronline.com	$179.00	x		
Evaluware	www.assistiveware.com	$125	x	x	

The SETT Framework: Critical Areas To Consider When Making Informed Assistive Technology Decisions
by Joy Zabala, http://sweb.uky.edu/~jszaba0/SETTintro.html

- The SETT Framework focuses on the student, the environment, the tasks, and the tools.

- It was produced to assist teams through a variety of activities needed to help students select, acquire, and use assistive technology devices and software.

- More information of the uses of SETT can be found at: www.connsensebulletin.com/resett3.html and www.ldonline.org/article/6399.

- Windows and Mac

- Free

WATI (The Wiscons Assistive Technology Initiative)
available from www.wati.org

- This program was designed to increase the capacity of school districts to provide assistive technology services by making training and technical assistance available to teachers, therapists, administrators, and parents throughout Wisconsin as they implement the assistive technology requirements of IDEA.
- This initiative provides manuals, assessment forms, self-assessment tools, children's stories, and examples of many successful applications.
- Many helpful free resources are available on their Web site in English and Spanish. Several include:
- Resource Guide for Teachers and Administrators about Assistive Technology (PDF)
- WATI Assessment — Forms only (PDF — 405Kb)
- AT Checklist — English (PDF — 498Kb)
- School Profile of Assistive Technology Services — A tool for school districts to analyze and improve their assistive technology services.
- Windows and Mac
- Free

COMPASS
by Koester Performance Research (KRP), www.kpronline.com

- Compass software measures the user's skills during computer interactions.
- It is designed to help clinical and educational professionals perform computer access evaluations with their clients and students.
- Skills assessed include keyboard and mouse use, navigation through menus, and switch use.
- It includes eight skill tests, covering text entry, and the use of pointing devices and switches.
- Each test has many configuration options to customize testing as needed. Compass collects speed and accuracy data during test performance and reports the results.
- Windows
- $179.00

EvaluWare
by AssistiveWare, www.assistiveware.com

- EvaluWare is a software program that was developed to identify the best computer access methods and ideal AAC setups for users with special needs.

- It combines several types of assessments into one package to identify the best settings and preferences for the user based on motor/access, looking, listening and other related skills.

- Motor/Access Skills are assessed through identifying the learner's appropriate input method and settings using a touch screen, mouse, switch, keyboard, or alternative pointer.

- Visual Skills are assessed through identifying the learner's ideal visual target size, number of items, and type of image.

- Listening Skills are assessed through identifying the learner's preferred voice, and type of feedback.

- This program also assesses the readiness of the user to use an on-screen keyboard and word prediction software.

- Windows and Mac

- $125.00

Stages Assessment Software
by Assistive Technology, Inc. www.assistivetech.com

- Stages Assessment Software helps identify a learner's skills and the ideal learning or assessment environment.

- The Stages framework gives a common language for reviewing learner progress. The seven stages are developmental in nature and are not age or grade specific.

- The software helps professionals select the ideal method for computer access using a mouse, touch screen, switch (1-switch auto or 2-switch step scanning), alternative keyboard (such as IntelliKeys), or pointer.

- Graphic representation such as photographs, drawings, symbols videos, or animations

- Feedback, which can be auditory, visual or combined, is appropriate for children, teens, or adults.

- Auditory, visual or combined prompts

- Activities to explore activities to introduce content or assess activities to test skills

- Full text-to-speech for writing activities

- Data Collection
- Stages All-in-One (1-7) with Stages Report Wizard is $795.00
- Stages All in One Children's Software Bundle $2,054.00
- Stages 1-7 Teen/Adult Software Bundle $2,054.00

Therapist and Client Attitudes and Expertise

Therapists and clients do not need to be computer savvy to benefit from the use of technology. The therapist's clinical expertise is much more predictive of success than his or her computer knowledge. Ideally, professionals and consumers who are new to the world of computers should learn from computer-literate therapists or friends to avoid some of the frustrations of using an unfamiliar technology.

To get the most out of this guide, therapists, clients, and others who act as "computer buddies" should have a basic knowledge of

- word processing,
- Internet access and basic search methods,
- e-mail use,
- procedure to load software, and
- rudimentary computer problem-solving solutions.

During the initial phase of computer use in treatment, it is helpful to find out the client's prior computer knowledge, interest, and use. During the first one or two treatment sessions using a computer, assess current abilities and comfort levels while observing general computer use. Computer skills that should be observed include

- using the mouse and keyboard,
- viewing text and images on the monitor,
- sequencing steps in a task,
- accessing and exiting programs, and
- loading software.

Backup Plan When Technology Fails

It's important to have a backup plan of more "conventional" therapy methods when the computer can't be used as planned. At one time or another, everyone will experience an unexpected computer glitch.

Software may not load properly if it is incompatible with the operating system or if there is insufficient memory. After an electrical storm, the system may need to be rebooted. Clients and therapists should have access to computer specialists to call for support as needed.

Attitude Toward Computers

We all encounter clients and professionals who do not like computers, who may have had negative experiences with them, or who just prefer methods of treatment that are more traditional. There are professionals who have heard that technology can improve therapy, but have tried it and found it to be more of a hindrance than a help. There are also professionals who have no computer experience and are reluctant to proceed in that direction. In the last case, some basic computer training or a mentorship with an experienced clinician might be an appropriate course of action. More computer skills may make entering the world of technology for therapy a more worthwhile and successful experience.

Once clients who had been hesitant start using the software, their fears are usually alleviated. A slower approach when working with people who are generally averse to using computers and technology is often more successful. In such cases, it may be helpful to begin with therapy methods that are more traditional and do not use computers. Gradually introduce computer-based tasks that are not threatening and might even be enjoyable.

For elderly clients who are reluctant to use computers, good entry points include viewing digital pictures of grandchildren, using talking photo albums, reading an online newspaper from a former place of residence (with a text reader if needed), incorporating personally relevant digital pictures and receiving and sending email. Software to improve particular communication or cognitive skills may be gradually added. Because of their prior exposure, younger clients might more often embrace the use of computers in therapy than might older clients.

People who have acquired communication and cognitive deficits often need step-by-step guidance and support to resume computer activities that they had been able to perform well before their injury. Often people who were confident computer users before a stroke or head injury try to resume computer activities that were once routine, but now are very difficult and they fail. Many individuals need help when they attempt to return to tasks such as the use of e-mail, word processing, and financial management to avoid frustration. Clinicians need to caution clients to go slowly when returning to previous technology-related activities.

Specialist Referrals

Professionals should clearly identify their areas of expertise and skill. When confronted with situations outside of those areas, it's in the best interest of the clients to help them explore alternative options with professionals who may be more skilled in that area. Many of the tools and resources reviewed in this guide may be helpful so that you can refer clients to associations and others who are experienced using products that are outside of your typical scope of practice.

Investment of Time and Money

Most professionals have budget constraints. To begin integrating technology into treatment, we often need hardware, software, and training. Professionals may be required to write proposals to obtain funds for hardware and software. Consumers want to spend their hard-earned money, on what will help them improve the most, but they may find it difficult to compare products and evaluate their potential utility. Many clinicians already have a computer and do not have the money to purchase additional software, adaptive hardware, and devices. Fortunately, computer use in treatment will probably increase your revenue.

Quite a bit can be accomplished with little monetary investment. The Internet provides a wealth of information and resources for free. Many of us already have items around the house or office, including computer programs, which can be used as effective therapy tools. Products such as Microsoft Windows, Microsoft Word, e-mail, calendars, maps, and clocks can help. In addition, free demo CDs, free downloads, free interactive Web sites, and organizations and online support groups can help in the treatment process. Many of these products are discussed throughout this guide. Chapter 16 reviews many free online interactive activities that can be used for treatment.

There are people who could benefit from using computers and other high-tech devices, but may not be able to afford them. In such cases, religious groups, local businesses, and community organizations may be able to help provide the necessary hardware and software.

Time Requirement

This guide will help you save time. It is organized to help you find helpful resources quickly for your clients. As mentioned previously, you may access suggested resources by selecting the setting in which you work, or by reading about particular communication or cognitive goal areas. There are also resources to help you quickly product treatment materials. Chapter 15 provides many resources for generating printed materials and ideas for using multi-media program in therapy. To access quickly the pages in this book that reference particular software programs, devices, or vendors, refer to the indexes at the back of the book.

Cool Tools — Top Picks

Many software products and devices on the market today are affordable and easy to use in therapy. These tools were produced for a wide variety of audiences— some for people with special communication or cognitive needs, others for people learning English as a second language, people with low vision, or mainstream society. In the hands of a creative and skilled therapist, these products can unlock the potential of many clients. The top picks mentioned below are discussed in detail later in this guide.

Many of these items were intended to help people who have difficulty with the following tasks:

- Language
- Voice
- Reading
- Thinking
- Remembering
- Speech
- Learning
- Writing
- Concentrating

There are also products developed for a more mainstream audience to make

- daily life easier, more enjoyable, and efficient at home, school, and work; and
- learning more fun and effective for individuals without diagnosed issues.

Software That Enables Computers To Read Aloud

Software that can read aloud is referred to as a "text reader" or "text-to-speech software." This technology often creates hope about potential technology treatment solutions. For many people, it also increases motivation. Text readers are reviewed in Chapter 12, "Treatment and Technology To Improve Reading Comprehension." The use of text-to-speech software is a great way to help improve the following tasks:

- Reading comprehension
- Reading speed
- Writing
- Proofreading

- Expressive communication
- Memory
- Auditory Processing
- Attention and concentration

When using text readers, you can select options to customize these tasks:

- Voice and rate of speech
- Font size and color
- Content that is read aloud
- Type of highlighting used

You can select the text that is read aloud from these places:

- E-mail
- A Web site
- A word processing document that is already in the computer
- A newspaper article, recipe, or other written document scanned into the computer
- Books presented in digital format
- PDF files

Software That Teaches English as a Second Language

Software developed to teach English as a second language is reviewed in Chapter 9, "Treatment and Technology To Improve Verbal Expression."

These products

- tend to be very interactive;
- focus on practical, everyday communication skills;
- include entertaining and educational games; and
- are reasonably priced.

Talking Photo Albums

Talking photo albums enable users to record the voice of a person, which can then be heard when pressing a nearby button. It can be easily customized to provide meaningful practice of relevant communication topics, to engage family members and friends in conversation, or to be used in treatment sessions. Talking photo albums are mentioned in Chapter 10, "Additional Tools and Resources To Improve Verbal Expression." Pictures can be placed in the following kinds of albums:

- Family
- Friends
- Places and people in the community to visit
- Items and rooms in the house
- Enjoyable activities

Adapted E-Mail and Internet Access

It's important for every client to be able to use e-mail and the Internet. E-mail is a great communication tool for maintaining social contacts and facilitating the assimilation of new information. They are described in Chapter 15, "Adapted E-mail, Search Engines, and Web Browsers." Adapted e-mail programs offer many helpful features such as

- pictures of people in the address book,
- the ability to "speak" messages as an alternative to typing them,
- the ability to have incoming messages read aloud, and
- large and simple icons and type.

Multi-Featured Software To Assist With Studying and Writing

Several programs on the market are helpful for struggling students and adults reentering the working world who need extra support with reading and writing. These products are reviewed in Chapter 13, "Treatment and Technology To Improve Written Expression."

These programs include the following features:

- Helping the user think of words with word prediction features
- Reducing the number of keystrokes needed for typing
- Easing the typing burden with preprogrammed phrases and sentences that can be accessed with abbreviations
- Help with reading speed and comprehension with text readers
- Assistance with proofreading by having the computer read aloud

- The ability to insert voice notes and text notes for future reference
- The ability to highlight information for later review, as well as to extract the highlighted material and place it in its own file
- Help with brainstorming ideas and formulating those ideas into a written narrative

New Handheld Technology To Help With Memory, Organization, and Communication

Handheld and wireless devices can be simplified and customized as needed to assist with memory, organization, and communication. With the help of a skilled clinician, they can provide new opportunities for people with communication and cognitive challenges to improve their overall quality of life. Many are discussed in Chapter 14, "Treatment and Technology To Improve Cognition and Memory."

The following devices are included:

- Cell phones
- Electronic organizers
- Pocket PCs
- Palms
- Digital cameras
- iPods and other MP3 players

Chapter 3:
Treatment Settings

It is challenging to decide what to purchase for the development or expansion of computer-based treatment for clients. The setting where the treatment takes place, occupation of the clinician, caseload guidelines, and level of clinical and computer expertise vary for each reader of this guide.

Education, rehabilitation, and wellness professionals may work in the following settings:

- Acute care hospitals

- Inpatient and outpatient rehabilitation centers

- Outpatient clinics

- Regular schools

- Learning centers

- Skilled nursing facilities, adult day-care centers, and retirement communities

- The client's home

- Work re-entry/vocational programs

- Special education schools

- Colleges and universities

Many different people who work in the fields of education and rehabilitation may benefit from reading this guide. They may work as the following types of professionals:

- Speech-language pathologists
- Assistive technology specialists
- Neuropsychologists
- Professors
- Social workers
- Administrators
- Teachers
- Special educators
- School counselors
- Technology coordinators
- Principals

- Occupational therapists
- Recreational therapists
- Psychologists
- Graduate students
- Case managers
- Tutors
- Reading specialists
- Learning disabilities teachers
- Media specialists
- Administrators
- Life coaches

They may have caseloads with which vary greatly from each other and may include:

- Children or adults

- People with developing abilities or degenerating abilities

- Severely impaired clients with little functional communication or high functioning clients with fluency or intelligibility issues

- A "niche" population with similar needs or a wide range of clients with many different challenges

- A large caseload or a small caseload

- Group therapy or individualized therapy

- Assessment or treatment

- Consultation with professionals or direct work with clients

- Short sessions or longer sessions

- Few sessions or many sessions

- Improving educational outcomes or improving rehabilitation outcomes

- Improving overall literacy or improving particular parameters of communication skills such as articulation, voice, or fluency

Also, the level of both clinical and computer expertise varies and may include:

- New graduate students with little experience vs. seasoned clinicians

- People who are not familiar with basic computer use vs. experienced computer users

- People who have used and attended courses on assistive and adaptive technology vs. people who have not been exposed to this approach to treatment

Top Picks for Getting Started Using Technology in Most Settings

The following is a list of suggested items that may be of value when starting to integrate technology into treatment. These products are also discussed in detail in chapters 9-17 of this guide. This list is meant to give you an overview to help you focus on materials that might be most appropriate for your situation. Each software program or adaptive device is also listed in the product index at the back of this book. There is also an index listing all vendors.

The programs listed together after each bullet are not identical, but overlap somewhat in their features. If your budget will not permit the purchase of these suggested items, it would be great if you could access the online demos or demo CDs of the programs to show to clients or try with them. There are also many helpful free online interactive programs, which are discussed in Chapter 17, "Games and Free Online Activities."

- Therasimplicity online subscription to generate practice materials. It is found at www.therasimplicity.com.

- Drill-and-practice CDs (for moderate to severe language goals) that are easy to get up and running quickly, so you can focus on helping clients with moderate and severe language deficits. These programs include Bungalow Software, Laureate Software, Attainment Software, and CHAT by Aphasia Therapy Products.

- A talking picture program (for expressive language), such as Clicker 5, IntelliTools Classroom Suite, Speaking Dynamically Pro, Writing With Symbols, or Picture Word Power

- ESL-oriented programs (targeting all language modalities), such as Learn to Speak English, Tell Me More!, Speak Now! English, World Talk English. or Rosetta Stone

- A program showing up-close mouth movement (for verbal expression), such as Speech Sounds on Cue or Speech Practice

- A comprehensive articulation-oriented program, such as Pronunciation Power or American Speech Sounds

- A text reader (to work on reading and writing), such as WordQ2, Universal Reader, Text Aloud or ReadPlease

- At least one program (to work on cognitive skills and memory), such as NeuroPsychOnline, Parrot Software, or Attention and Memory

- A subscription to adapted newspapers, such as News-2-You or Current Events

- E-mail access to mainstream programs, such as AOL and Outlook, and one adapted e-mail program, such as ICanEmail or Springdoo

- At least one single-level talking device, such as a Talking Photo Album, GoTalk, or Listen to Me

- A few non-technology items to help with word retrieval and communication of basic needs, such as the Oxford Picture Dictionary, Daily Communicator, calendars, maps, clocks, cards, and games

- Information from www.ittsguides.com or Chapter 17 in this guide about Web sites for online support and information grouped by disability

- Listings of Web sites or sample catalogs of vendors who sell items to assist with daily living, many of which are listed at www.ittsguides.com Some of these include the following Web sites:
  - www.abledata.com, assistive technology information, 800-227-0216
  - www.alimed.com, medical and ergonomic products, 800-225-2610
  - www.enablemart.com, helpful technology-related products, 888-640-1999
  - www.interactivetherapy.com, speech and hearing products for stroke survivors, 800-253-5111

Acute Care

Professionals who work in acute care hospital settings have a unique set of challenges. The average length of an individual's stay has become increasingly brief. Most clinicians have only a few visits with patients. There is little time to get a good grasp of the client's comprehensive needs after discharge and the potential benefits technology may be able to play in the improvement of communication and cognition.

Our professional roles have changed:

- Occupational therapy (OT) sessions tend to focus on the use of upper extremities and the activities of daily living.
- Case managers now focus on discharge plans and case coordination.
- Speech-language pathologists focus on the following issues:
  - Evaluating and managing dysphagia (swallowing disorders)
  - Counseling family members of client's who have communication and cognitive deficits
  - Discharge planning for continued speech therapy rehabilitation efforts after discharge
  - Providing a means of communication for individuals who are unable to communicate
  - Initiating a few sessions of therapy to evaluate, improve, and compensate for communication and cognitive abilities

Computer-based therapy, during the few sessions that are available with inpatients in acute care, is not generally recommended. However, clinicians, administrators, and care managers can have a significant impact on the lives of people with communication and cognitive challenges by making resources known to the clients and their families. Knowledge is power. The software, devices, and Web sites reviewed in this guide may be a way for patients to improve their skills outside of the limited, inpatient treatment, time framework. The dedicated communication devices (with or without environmental controls) and communication boards and books can provide a way for people to communicate when their medical condition makes talking difficult.

Top Picks for Getting Started With Technology in Acute Care Settings

Although the focus of treatment in acute care is not on the use of computers for therapy, the following is a list of suggested items that may be of value in addition to the "Top Picks for Getting Started Using Technology in Most Settings" listed earlier in this chapter. As mentioned earlier, please refer to the product index or vendor index at the end of this guide to locate quickly more information about resources.

Critical Communicator (Revised)
by Interactive Therapeutics, www.interactivetherapy.com

- This is a word-and-picture communication board. Basic care concepts are provided in an easy-to-use menu format.

- It is appropriate for use with people in critical care settings such as ICU, trauma units, emergency departments, specialized ventilator units, post-surgery areas, long-term care, home health, and hospices.

- There are twenty-five communication boards per package, and they are available in English or Spanish for $23.00.

Critical Communicator for Kids
by Interactive Therapeutics, www.interactivetherapy.com

- This child-friendly word-and-picture communication board includes foods, activities, and toys, as well as a pain scale and other needs.

- This board can be used to assist family and staff to interact with children who need help communicating on a temporary basis.

- It's helpful in post-surgery areas, emergency rooms, intensive care, and trauma and specialized units.

- It's printed on heavy 81/2 × 11-inch card stock in a menu format.

- A pack of twenty-five copies is available in English or Spanish for $23.00.

Vidatak E-Z Board
by Vidatak, www.vidatak.com

- The Vidatak E-Z Board, an 11 × 17-inch preprinted dry-erase board, is a fourth-generation product that has recently been redesigned based on clinical research findings.

- It is available in fifteen different languages.

- $16.50

Skilled Nursing Facilities, Adult Day-Care Providers, and Retirement Communities

Personal computers can provide a source of enjoyment as well as help people in long-term living situations improve and maintain communication and cognition. Residents in skilled nursing facilities and retirement communities as well as participants in adult day-care programs can be seen for individual therapy or group therapy that integrates the use of technology. The challenge to the professional is creating engaging and mentally stimulating exercises that seniors will enjoy and continue to practice. The computer can serve as a therapeutic and rehabilitative tool, as well as a form of social and educational enrichment. Newly emerging technologies have made these tools affordable.

It is a well-known fact that mental stimulation is imperative for the elderly. Incorporating computer use into programming has many advantages:

- Technology can help people facilitate communication, access information, explore options for entertainment and learning, and promote overall independence.

- As the elderly population increases, communication, and cognitive rehabilitation professionals can play an important role in meeting the diverse social, recreational, and intellectual needs of the elderly with the help of computers and technology.

- Once candidates have been seen by a communication and cognitive specialist for a few sessions to obtain a brief assessment and conduct a trial of cognitive and communicative retraining, they can benefit from working on their own with the assistance of computer buddies, volunteers, or aides.

Computer labs should be available to all residents or participants. Specialized individualized support needs to be given to those who have cognitive and communicative issues. Small, hands-on classes can be offered on particular topics of interest or to help reach particular goals.

Areas of computer-related interest may include:

- Regular and adapted e-mail programs

- Word processing with accessibility options

- Text readers for improved reading comprehension and writing

- Software to help keep the brain sharp

- Software to help improve particular communication skills or address cognitive weaknesses, such as impaired memory and word retrieval

- Games for cognitive stimulation and enjoyment

- Videophones to stay in touch with family and see them while talking

- Use of the Internet to research treatment options, medications, and products and to promote self-advocacy

- Digital photography

- E-books

- Digital greeting cards

- Review of Web sites, chat rooms, newsgroups, and listservs pertaining to particular hobbies and interests

It is not the role of the communication or cognitive specialist to create computer labs or provide basic computer training to participants. There are computer specialists and administrators who are trained in this area. However, communication specialists should be used to assist in the selection of hardware and software for computer labs and to heighten awareness of what can be offered to help people stimulate the areas of reading, writing, talking, listening, remembering, and thinking.

Computer access can greatly improve the overall perception of a facility's ability to meet the needs of its clients or residents and promote their wellbeing. There is a slow, but steady trend toward offering computers and Internet access to the geriatric population.

The Client's Home

Therapy in the home offers both advantages and disadvantages:

Advantages of Home-Based Treatment

- Clients may feel more comfortable in their familiar everyday surroundings.

- It's often easier to focus on practical solutions to specific issues in the home.

- Professionals can assist with modifications and customizations to the computer and living environment.

- Training can easily take place with caregivers so that new techniques and assignments can be practiced to facilitate learning and carryover.

Disadvantages of Home-Based Treatment

- Clients may be distracted with phone calls, household chores, and interruptions by family members.

- The environment may be cluttered or otherwise not conducive to focused treatment.

- It's a burden to carry a computer, software, and other materials to use with the client at home prior to working on their own system—if they have one.

- The client will need to wait until the next session if the clinician wants to try using something that wasn't brought to the home.

Notebook or Tablet Computer

- It's helpful to have a notebook or tablet computer loaded with software to use with a client in his or her home.

- For the first few sessions, make adaptive computer equipment available as needed.

Home Computer

- Provide contact information for professionals who can assist the family with setting up high-speed Internet access, making sure there is sufficient computer memory and that the computer is virus-free, establishing home wireless networks, and providing computer maintenance and virus protection if they do not already have someone who can provide that service.

- Encourage family members and caregivers who are unfamiliar with computers to take a basic course or learn from readily available DVDs, CDs, and books.

- Encourage the client who is not experienced with computer use to enlist the help of a computer buddy who is well versed with word processing, loading software, backing up documents, and troubleshooting when something goes wrong with the computer.

- Use a contract that releases you from liability for damage to the client's computer during treatment sessions. It could be disastrous if a client's financial records or other important documents were infected with a virus or accidentally deleted. It is advised that legal counsel be consulted to make sure that the contract/release form is adequate.

- Carefully consider the selection of programs to load onto the client's computer. We first try out programs on our computer to determine their effectiveness with the client.

Suggestions To Make the Home Environment Conducive To Learning

- Clear clutter from the area so that the user has a clear workspace and storage space.

- Make sure that the user's positioning and seating are ergonomically appropriate with good support.

- Eliminate distractions such as the TV or radio.

- Use favorable lighting.

- Place the computer in an easily accessible location to promote the likelihood of practice between sessions.

Rehabilitation and Outpatient Clinics

To provide the highest quality of treatment, computers and technology must play an integral role in both inpatient and outpatient rehabilitation.

Intensity of Treatment

Quite a bit of literature supports the notion that intensive therapy produces greater outcomes. Specific references can be found in Chapter 8, "Supportive Research." The computer empowers clients to increase the intensity of their practice.

Home Practice Programs

Specific instructions for individual practice as well as the software with which to practice are essential components of an effective therapy program.

Clients who are in the initial stages of rehabilitation often have limited endurance and many demands on their time from different rehabilitation disciplines and doctors' appointments. As endurance improves and clients settle into a routine, one to two hours on assignments a day is suggested to maximize progress.

Schools

Benefits of Technology in the School Setting

Parents are increasingly taking an active role in exploring potential treatment options for their children. They are learning more about the use of assistive technology to help their children become independent at home, in the classroom, at work, and in society. They expect the schools to provide the supportive services to make it happen.

Clinicians and administrators in the school setting need to familiarize themselves with a variety of technology-oriented options to assist students in reaching their full potential. Educators can use technology to help a wide variety of students. Integrating technology into the school day is helpful for students with the following characteristics or needs:

- Have language and learning challenges and disabilities
- Are English language learners
- Are gifted learners
- Are at risk for failure

Technology can be used to assist with these tasks:

- Following directions
- Learning grammar and punctuation
- Speaking more clearly
- Enhancing vocabulary
- Practicing writing
- Studying for exams
- Improving spelling and vocabulary
- Researching on the Internet
- Improving organization, sequencing, and reasoning

The role of a school-based clinician today is very different from in the past. The following statements are true of most of today's school systems:

- Caseloads are larger.
- Children are typically seen for individual therapy only if their communication or cognitive deficit has a negative impact on academic performance.

- The content of therapy sessions is more curriculum-based.

- The pullout model is most common for students with articulation/phonology, voice, or fluency disorders.

- Many therapists spend more time in the classroom and group treatment than with individual therapy.

- Language-enrichment services are often provided with larger group instruction or co-taught with the classroom teacher.

- Consultation with other educational personnel and parents is often used to provide services indirectly.

- Speech-language pathologists are most often members of a school team. These teams provide consultation, evaluation, and training for students with augmentative communication needs due to severe speech impairments.

Increasingly, computers are found in regular as well as special education classrooms. Students and teachers use technology for a variety of purposes:

- Going online for research projects.

- Obtaining supplemental help with standardized tests and homework.

- Typing and printing essays.

- Getting graphics for projects.

- Staying involved in the social network.

- Providing distance education and support.

New technologies continue to emerge that lure children into the world of technology. In an age of instant messaging, iPods, Web journals, social networking Internet sites, and the reliance of the educational system on the use of the Internet and technology, many children use computer-based products multiple times a day. Often, students who have communication and cognitive deficits have not kept up with these technology trends, which places them at an educational and social disadvantage.

Teachers and therapists in schools are now integrating technology into the educational process. The school districts tend to make decisions regarding which software to purchase and use in the schools. With the help of this guide, clinicians will be better able to influence these decisions and help select the best software and hardware to help students with communication and cognitive challenges.

Evaluation Protocols

Several protocols are available online for professionals to use to develop an understanding of the needs of students in the classroom environment. They offer a way to systematically evaluate whether the student does or does not complete a set of tasks that the staff feels should be completed, and offer a framework from which to being the selection of assistive technology solutions. The two most popular frameworks used in the school setting are referred to as SETT or WATI.

Title	Web Site	Price	PC	Mac
The SETT Framework	http://sweb.uky.edu/~jszaba0/SETTintro.html	Free	x	x
WATI	www.WATI.com	Free	x	x
AT Profile	http://assistivetech.com	$150.00		

The SETT framework: Critical Areas to Consider When Making Informed Assistive Technology Decisions
by Joy Zabala, http://sweb.uky.edu/~jszaba0/SETTintro.html

- The SETT Framework focuses on the student, the environment, the tasks, and the tools. It was produced to assist teams through a variety of activities needed to help students select, acquire, and use assistive technology devices and software.

- The integration of the technology into everyday routines at school is often the most difficult challenge faced in the schools. Repeated use of this framework is a helpful tools to help teams collaborate to support the AT user. More information of the uses of SETT can be found at these sites:
http://www.connsensebulletin.com/resett3.html
http://www.ldonline.org/article/6399.

WATI (The Wisconsin Assistive Technology Initiative)
available at www.wati.org

- This program was designed to increase the capacity of school districts to provide assistive technology services by making training and technical assistance available to teachers, therapists, administrators, and parents throughout Wisconsin. The initiative has developed manuals, assessment forms, self-assessment tools, children's stories, and examples of many successful applications.

- Many helpful free resources are available on their Web site in English and Spanish, including these:

- Resource Guide for Teachers and Administrators about Assistive Technology (PDF)

- WATI Assessment - Forms only (PDF - 405Kb)

- AT Checklist - English (PDF - 498Kb)

AT Profile
by Assistive Technology, http://assistivetech.com

- This new tool helps educators and clinicians keep track of the AT needs, successes, and progress of their students.

- This Profile identifies AT tools, tracks the success of each one, and notes the specific settings needed to ensure success.

- Information can then be incorporated into the student's IEP. Checklist categories include: communication abilities, grid preferences, hearing, vision, mobility, seating and positioning, writing, educational strategies for reading and math, study strategies, computer access and preferences, recreation/leisure, activities of daily living, educational software, hardware/devices and supports, and an equipment tracking system.

- 10 booklets and CD cost $150.00

There is a growing trend toward training teachers and special educators in the use of technology to improve the effectiveness of their teaching and to meet the learning needs of students.

Assistive Technology: A Way to Differentiate Instruction for Students with Disabilities`
National Professional Resources
http://www.nprinc.com

- This CD features Dr. Brian Friedlander as he visits in schools with teachers and students, selects appropriate solutions to their special learning, and oversees their progress.

- $139.00

More information on this topic can be found on the following Web sites:

- Education World, www.education-world.com

- Georgia Project for Assistive Technology, www.gpat.org

- International Society for Technology in Education, www.iste.org

- Preparing Tomorrow's Teachers to Use Technology, www.pt3.org

- Project Participate, www.projectparticipate.org

- Read WriteThink.org, www.readwritethink.org

- Tech for Learning Consortium, www.techforlearning.com

Mainstream Preschool and Elementary School Software

After a comprehensive evaluation, it is helpful to show parents how to provide supplementary practice toward speech goals with mainstream software and Web-based resources. These programs are typically very reasonably priced, interactive, and entertaining. One quick way to locate mainstream software that is organized by grade, age, or subject is by going to www.amazon.com and selecting the most helpful search method.

Several Web sites provide helpful reviews of this software:

- **Children's Software Online**, www.childrenssoftwareonline.com

- **All Star Review**, www.allstarreview.com

- **SuperKids**, www.superkids.com

Many Web sites sell pediatric software:

- **Software for Schools**, www.NationalSchoolProducts.com

- **Amazon**, www.amazon.com

- **Kids Click**, www.kidsclick.com

- Selectsoft Publishing, www.selectsoft.com

- **Cyber City Software**, www.cybercitysoftware.com

Mainstream preschool and elementary school software and electronic tools can be used to help children who have literacy issues. Here are the top picks:

- **JumpStart Software** by Knowledge Adventure,
  www.knowledgeadventure.com

- **Humongous Entertainment Software,** available at many of the previously listed Web sites, such as Putt Putt and Freddi Fish

- **LeapFrog products,** www.leapfrog.com, such as the FLY Pentop Computer and LeapPad electronic learning toys

- **Riverdeep Software,** www.Riverdeep.com, such as The Edmark House Series, Thinkin' Things, and the Reader Rabbit Series. Riverdeep is now the parent company of Learning Company and Edmark.

- **Scholastic Software,** www.scholastic.com, such as Thinking Reader and Reading for Meaning

- Sunburst Technology , www.sunburst.com

Specialized Software for Students

Software that is produced to target specific communication and cognitive goals for children is often more expensive than mainstream products, but focuses more directly on particular aspects of speech, language, and cognition. Many of these programs are discussed in Chapters 9-14. The following programs are included here in the schools section because they promote overall literacy.

Title	Web Site
Janelle Publications	www.janellepublications.com
Laureate Learning System	www.laureatelearning.net
LinguiSystems	www.linguisystems.com
Talking Finger	www.readwritetype.com
Time4Learning	www.time4learning.com

Janelle Publications
available at www.janellepublications.com

- Janelle Publications offers a wide variety of software to facilitate treatment for improving language, pragmatics, articulation and phonology, phonics, and literacy with children.

Laureate Learning Systems
available at www.laureatelearning.net

- Laureate Learning offers a wide variety of software for training: vocabulary, expressive language, categorization, syntax, auditory discrimination and processing, concept development, functional language, and reading and spelling.

LinguiSystems
available from www.linguisystems.com

- LinguiSystems offers Basic Concept Pictures Interactive Software, the No-Glamour Series, and the Autism and PDD Series.

Talking Fingers, Inc
available at www.readwritetype.com

- Read, Write & Type is a program that merges the teaching of phonics-based reading skills with typing.

- In the Read, Write & Type Learning System (steps 1 -7), characters help children foil a plot of a villain through 40 levels, building hundreds of animated sentences and stories as they go.

- In the Spaceship Challenge CD (steps 8-12), children engage in skill-strengthening games. Children learn to hear the individual sounds in words, and associate each sound with a letter and a finger stroke on the keyboard.

- Parents and teachers can customize the program for different reading levels and proficiency targets.

- Mac and Windows.

- The Home Edition is $79.00. A curriculum pack is $289.00

Time4Learning
available at www.time4learning.com

- This company offers a learning system that builds and reinforces reading, writing, and math skills.

- It is an interactive online environment that mixes educational lessons with learning games.

- It can be used as core or supplementary curriculum.

- Children progress at their own rate using multi-sensory learning that helps each learning style.

- The cost is $19.95 a month for online subscription.

Software Offering Curriculum-Based Support

The following Web sites offer assistance with training, as well as many downloadable programs that focus on integrating speech therapy lessons into the general education curriculum in areas such as science, English, and social studies.

- www.intellitools.com
- www.donjohnston.com
- www.cricksoft.com
- www.quickmind.net

Word Processing Software

Microsoft Word and other word processing programs offer a wide variety of features and accessibility options that are helpful to kids with and without communication and learning issues. Each of these products offers unique features, such as word prediction, word banks, text-to-speech, voice recognition, advanced spelling, and grammar checking, and study tools. These programs are discussed in more detail in Chapters 12, "Treatment and Technology To Improve Reading Comprehension," or Chapter 13, "Treatment and Technology To Improve Written Expression."

- **Kurzweil 3000**, www.kurzweiledu.com
- **Read &Write GOLD**, www.texthelp.com
- **WYNN Wizard**, www.freedomscientific.com
- **WordQ 2 and SpeakQ**, www.wordq.com
- **Talking Word Processor**, www.readingmadeeasy.com

Multimedia and Current Events Software

Children who have special needs, as well as those who don't, will benefit from a wide variety of media. Communication and cognitive tasks can be integrated into creating works of art with a variety of drawing tools, photos and video, text, sounds, and special effects. Please refer to Chapter 16, "Multi-Media Programs and Generating Printed Treatment Materials."

Visual-Based Support

Graphic organizers are helpful tools for organizing ideas before writing for kids with and without special needs. Please refer to the Chapter 13, "Treatment and Technology To Improve Written Expression."

Other Tools That May Be Helpful for Students

- Specialized software has been developed for handheld technology to assist students with memory impairments. This technology is becoming increasingly popular in school environments. Examples can be found at www.ablelinktech.com and www.brainaid.com.

- Search engines have been produced to help students learn and recall facts. www.askforkids.com is a site that provides many news resources for kids, books for study help in academic areas and a variety of fun and games.

- A dictation service for students was developed for children who struggle with the tasks of writing a paper. More information can be found at www.idictate.com. The user can dictate any document using a telephone, fax machine, or dictation device, and then receive the completed job back for editing via e-mail within a day.

Helpful Web Sites for Advocacy, Therapy, Homework and Information for Students

Refer to Chapter 17, "Games and Free Online Interactive Activities," for additional suggestions.

- **Academic Info** (www.academicinfo.net) — Provides many links to high quality educational resources. It is an online subject directory of over 25,000 educational resources for high school and college students as well as a directory of online degree programs and admissions test preparation resources (SAT, GRE, LSAT, MCAT, GMAT, USMLE, TOEFL). They offer timely news and analysis of critical current events.

- **Literactive** (www.literactive.com) — Provider of online reading materials for preschool, kindergarten, and first-grade students. The program is composed of readers that are provided with varying levels of difficulty, comprehensive phonic activities, and a wealth of supplemental reading materials that gradually develop a child's reading skills in a sequential and enjoyable manner. The material is available free from this site.

- **Scholastic** (www.scholastic.com/kids/homework/organizer.htm) — Offers many hints and tools to help students get organized. It's very appealing and colorful.

- **Study Buddy** (www.studybuddy.com) — A free interactive Web site to help with homework. Users type a question in StudyBuddy search and answers are displayed. People enter their grade level and browse through thousands of articles on hundreds of topics, all designed to help with homework. This site is sponsored by AOL.

- **TASH** (www.tash.org) — An organization that provides innovative educational strategies; cutting-edge research; and grassroots, personal, and collaborative advocacy.

- **Transition** (www.ed.gov/about/offices/list/ocr/transition.html) — A U.S. Department of Education resource for students with disabilities preparing for postsecondary education.

- **WebGrammar** (www.webgrammar.com) — A free online resource to help with writing. There are dictionaries, glossaries, grammar basics, grammar tips, idioms, homonyms, and additional resources to help with writing.

- **Wrightslaw** (www.wrightslaw.com) — A Web resource for parents, educators, and advocates for children with disabilities.

- **Woodbine House** (www.woodbinehouse.com) — A publisher specializing in books about children with special needs.

College and University Settings

Computers are everywhere in secondary academic settings. They are found throughout campuses. They are in the dorms, instructional computer labs, libraries, and offices. Equal access to education is linked to computer access. The use of computers with voice output, large screen displays, and other adaptive technologies is necessary so that students, faculty, and staff with disabilities can have equal access to the use of technology. Library electronic card catalogs, online course schedules, assignments, and social networks are now technology oriented.

Students who relied on others to take notes can now use a portable computer with voice-recognition software that enables them to take their own notes. Text readers, word predictors, study helpers, spelling and grammar checkers, handhelds and other computer-based systems can all be used to assist people whose disabilities make it difficult to communicate, read, write, organize, and analyze information.

Interactive whiteboards are becoming commonplace in academic settings and can transform the learning process. An interactive whiteboard is a dry-erase whiteboard writing surface that can capture writing electronically. Interactive applications are in demand for educators and clinicians who want to involve their students and clients in learning with technology. They are largely taking over the use of blackboards and whiteboards.

Interactive whiteboards work as a large computer screen by projecting the computer image onto the board via an external projector. The computer can actually be controlled via the board; a digital projector displays the computer images where they can be seen and manipulated. Users can control software both from the computer and from the board. By using a finger as a mouse, the teacher or student can run applications directly from the board. Another user at the computer can also have input. Any notes or drawings can then be saved or printed. There are three different types of boards with different ways of controlling the computer: electromagnetic, touch-sensitive, and infrared.

The interactive whiteboard has the following qualities:

- It is ideal for presentations.
- It allows students to work together on activities.
- Sessions can be recorded.

- Notes may be printed for immediate distribution or transcription, or they can be e-mailed and read online.

- Zoom features are helpful for individuals with visual impairments.

- Clients can practice the material at home.

- Brief instructional blocks can be recorded for review. The exact presentation can be viewed that occurred in the session with the audio input.

- The board can accommodate different learning styles. Tactile learners can benefit from touching and marking at the board. Auditory learners can have the class discussion, and visual learners can see what is taking place as it develops at the board.

- It's a colorful tool. Marking can be customized both in the pen and in the highlighter features to display a number of different colors.

More information can be found at these Web sites:

- SMART Board, www.smarttech.com
- Mimio, www.mimio.com

Return to Work and Volunteer Positions

Returning to work after a head injury or stroke, or finding a job for a person with language and learning issues is challenging. Careful preparation and the provision of support are critical.

It's beneficial for communication and cognitive specialists to collaborate with vocational rehabilitation counselors to help people with disabilities comprehend both their strengths and limitations. Clients must develop an understanding of the impact of their challenges, as well as how to compensate for them. The use of technology can be instrumental in establishing a smooth transition from rehabilitation to work or a volunteer position.

The Americans with Disabilities Act (ADA), which is described at www.ada.gov and www.eeoc.gov/policy/ada.html, requires an employer with fifteen or more employees to provide reasonable accommodation for employees with disabilities unless doing so would cause "undue hardship." According to the ADA, "a reasonable accommodation is any change in the work environment or in the way a job is performed that enables a person with a disability to enjoy equal employment opportunities." More information on the interpretation of this act is at www.eeoc.gov/facts/accommodation.html.

The technological hardware and software described in this guide are examples of reasonable accommodations that provide solutions for people who have communication and cognitive deficits and who are returning to work.

Reasonable Accommodations for People With Communication and Cognitive Impairments

To help the transition to work be successful, clinicians can assist by making the following changes:

- Help assess work-related activities and restructure or modify tasks as needed with frequent rest periods.

- Set up computer-based supports to help with reading, writing, and analysis of material with assistive technology. Examples include text readers, talking word processors, and communication systems.

- Establish strategies to promote well-organized and efficient work routines.

- Train others at the work site to communicate effectively with the client and raise their awareness of disability-related issues.

- Help clients find volunteer positions prior to return to work to practice effective strategies for successful reentry into the working world.

Technology That May Help With Reading and Writing Work-Related Responsibilities

Refer to Chapter 12, "Treatment and Technology to Improve Reading Comprehension," and Chapter 13, "Treatment and Technology to Improve Written Expression," to learn more about the use of text readers, word prediction software and talking word processors.

Technology That May Help With Communication, Organization, and Memory at Work

Refer to Chapter 14, Treatment and Technology to Improve Cognition and Memory," to learn more about sscheduling and brainstorming software, adapted e-mail, videophones and handhelds with Pocket PCs and Palm operating systems.

Helpful Web Sites and Other Resources To Help People Enter the Workforce

- The Job Accommodation Network (JAN), a service of the Office of Disability Employment Policy (ODEP), http://www.dol.gov/dol/topic/disability/jobaccommodation s.htm

- Work Re-Entry at the Brain Injury Resource Center, www.headinjury.com/jobs.htm

- Office of Special Education and Rehabilitative Services, www.ed.gov/about/offices/list/osers

- Diversity World, www.diversityworld.com

- The Learning Edge and Northern Edge, http://www.nwt.literacy.ca/northernedge/NorthernEdgeThumbnail. html

The Learning Edge and the Northern Edge are online literacy newspapers from Canada designed for adult literacy students. These Web-based resources are interactive and easy to use, with activities for adult learners using Flash. The Learning Edge has a new edition, with a focus on finding employment. Activities include networking, using the Internet to find jobs, and sample interview questions, as well as stories from learners about their work.

Volunteering

It's often helpful for people who would like to join or rejoin the paid working world to first pursue a volunteer position. These are two helpful Web sites:

- www.volunteer.gov
- www.volunteermatch.org

Chapter 4:
10 Scenarios and Technology Treatment Tips

As you read this guide, you may feel exhilarated by the possibilities for more creative treatment sessions or you may feel that you are on a whirlwind tour of an endless array of resources with which to help your clients. There is so much information it is often hard to know where to begin. In Chapter 3, software and other resources were listed to help you learn to initiate or expand the use of technology based on your work setting. This chapter offers guidance by describing several initial considerations for the use of technology based on the challenges and diagnosis of the client, student, or patient. Ideas are presented to help you get started in your quest to figure out which software, adaptive hardware, and other resources might help. Each scenario assumes that a comprehensive evaluation has already been completed and that functional goals for each person have been established.

Please keep in mind that the number of potential scenarios is limitless. The scenarios presented in this chapter offer a mere glimpse of the potential treatment solutions technology can offer individuals. Each person is different and every therapist has a unique treatment style and approach. The suggestions in this chapter were written to stimulate ideas and get the ball rolling. Each rehabilitation and education professional will adapt and change the ideas to meet the needs of particular situations. Of course, each client will respond differently to treatment and new paths will form for the implementation of new products as treatment progresses.

In each scenario, chapters in this guide that are predominately helpful for the given situation are listed, and the pages where products and vendors can be found are located in the Product Index and Vendor Indexes at the back of the guide.

As you become more familiar with certain products, you will more easily begin to adapt the use of software and other resources and use them in different ways with different clients. This is not an exact science. The best method for integrating technology into treatment is not set in stone. Working with each person requires creativity, practice, and quite a lot of trial and error to determine the optimal solution.

In every scenario, it is essential for professionals to do the following tasks:

- First, complete a comprehensive assessment to determine appropriate functional goals for treatment.

- Continue to provide traditional therapy.

- Empower family members with information and support by referring them to national organizations and associations. Helpful Web sites and discussion groups are presented in Chapter 19, "Online Support, Information and Discussion Groups."

- Keep up with the literature and continue to explore how new research and clinical findings and products can be used in treatment to improve client satisfaction.

- Show clients how they can work more on their own to reach their goals.

- Connect with other professionals in your field or in other fields to provide the highest quality of treatment possible. Chapter 19 lists online helpful resources by profession.

Scenarios

1. An adult in rehabilitation had a stroke.

2. An adult is not performing work duties well after a head injury.

3. An adult has gradual memory decline.

4. An adult has Parkinson's Disease and intelligibility issues.

5. An adult has advanced ALS and requires augmentative and assistive communication devices (AAC.)

6. An adult is in an acute care hospital because of a ruptured aneurysm.

7. An adult has difficulty making himself understood because of a foreign accent.

8. A child has speech that is difficult to understand because of apraxia.

9. A child is not performing well in school after a concussion.

10. A child has language, learning, and literacy challenges.

Scenario 1: Dealing With a Stroke

A 45-year-old outpatient who had a stroke is now in therapy to improve moderate communication and cognitive deficits.

Technology Tips

- Start out using Aphasia Tutor 1 Out: Loud and Aphasia Tutor 2 Out: Loud by Bungalow software to get a feel for computer use, reading, writing, talking, and listening abilities. Use of the software can be integrated into the actual treatment session to help pinpoint where to begin therapy.

- Focus on setting up clients with software that they can use at home to speed up progress. Loan them the Bungalow trial CD that can be purchased for $9.40. Suggest the programs to load on a home computer and which options should be selected. They can practice them following your guidance and then purchase the program that they found to be the most helpful.

- Try using some of the Attainment Company software that offers clear pictures with easy to follow instructions. Specific programs and pages with information are listed in the Vendor Index at the back of this guide. There are great demos for the Attainment Company software that clients can use at home, and then buy if desired.

- Use WordQ, Universal Reader or TextAloud to work on reading and typing in functional situations such as e-mail and exploring Web sites of interest.

- Explore the many therapy resources at therasimplicity.com or other programs to generate printed materials for independent practice. More information can be found in Chapter 16, "Multi-Media Programs and Generating Printed Treatment Materials."

- Try the online subscription to Parrot Software and figure out which of the many programs will be most effective. Another person or "computer buddy" might be needed to help the user find the appropriate lesson to practice and set up the options during home practice. Parrot software is especially helpful for people with moderate level cognitive and communication challenges.

- Try using software that provides words in natural settings and can be used for a variety of communication and cognitive tasks, such as the My House software by Laureate Learning or Looking for Words by Attainment Company and Talk Now! American English by EuroTalk. These are discussed in Chapter 9, "Treatment and Technology to Improve Verbal Expression."

- Additional suggestions can be found in the Rehabilitation and Outpatient Clinics section of Chapter 3, "Treatment Settings."

Scenario 2: Dealing With a Head Injury

A successful businessman is becoming increasingly forgetful and less productive at work after a head injury. He fears losing his job.

Technology Tips

- Analyze his work-related responsibilities and figure out where he needs to improve and support his skills.

- Create supportive routines and organizational strategies to maximize success. Suggestions are listed in Chapter14, "Treatment and Technology To Improve Cognition and Memory."

- Review assistive reading technology such as Word Q that can help speed up processing and retention of information and help with word retrieval. These tools are discussed in Chapter 12, "Treatment and Technology To Improve Reading Comprehension."

- Try out assistive writing technology such as the Ultimate Talking Dictionary by Premiere Assistive Technology to help with word retrieval, and brainstorming software, such as Inspiration by Inspiration to help with organizing written narrative. These items are reviewed in Chapter 13, "Treatment and Technology to Improve Written Expression."

- Introduce this client to handheld organizers which can help with word retrieval, managing "to do" lists, and remembering and planning appointments. These suggestions are also reviewed in Chapter 14.

- Show this client software that he can practice to improve cognitive skills such as NeuroPsychOnline, Brainbuilder and Brain Age. These programs are discussed in Chapter 14.

- Connect the family to online resources mentioned in Chapter 19, "Online Support, Information, and Discussion Groups."

- Work with people in the work setting, so that they understand the nature of the deficits and learn strategies that might help with productivity.

Scenario 3: Dealing With Gradual Memory Decline

An elderly woman who lives alone at home spends most of her time watching TV and shows gradual memory loss. Her children want to know what they can do to help her keep her "brain sharp."

Technology Tips

- Encourage her children and caregivers to use items such as calendars, maps, and talking photo albums to facilitate communication and establish daily routines. These suggestions are discussed in Chapter 14, "Treatment and Technology To Improve Cognition and Memory."

- To foster interactions with others, encourage the family to play games, which are reviewed in Chapter 17, "Games and Free Online Interactive Activities."

- Suggest that the family try some of the adapted e-mail programs such as ICanEmail by RJ Cooper. Adapted e-mail can be found in Chapter 15.

- Encourage the family to search for community-based programs to offer structured stimulation such as adult day care or assistive living communities.

- Offer ideas to a person who can play the role of her "computer buddy" and provide assistance with activities such as producing online greeting cards, and reviewing a weekly News-2-You newspaper available from News-2-You.com. This online newspaper, which can be printed out, provides weekly written current events with picture support to review as well as other activities that relate to the written information.

- Discuss options with the family for purchasing a simplified cell phone, so that she can call as needed when out alone. These are reviewed in Chapter 10, "Additional Tools and Resources To Improve Verbal Expression."

- Review the sections in Chapter 2, "Treatment Settings," which discusses ideas for therapy in the client's home.

Scenario 4: Dealing With Parkinson's Disease

A woman has Parkinson's Disease and is difficult to understand.

Technology Tips

- Try devices such as talking amplifiers and the Speech Enhancer to help provide speech that is more intelligible. These are discussed in Chapter 10, "Additional Tools and Resources To Improve Verbal Expression."

- Use software such as Sights 'N Sounds by Bungalow Software or American Speech Sounds by Speech Com to focus on the remediation of specific speech sound production.

- Print out worksheets for lists to practice speech production with using therasimplicity.com or use other resources from which is it easy to generate printed practice materials. Suggestions are listed in Chapter 16, "Multi-Media Programs and Generating Printed Treatment Materials."

- Try using a text reader such as Universal Reader by Premiere Assistive Technology or WordQ2 by Quillsoft to practice reading aloud from interesting Web sites, e-mails or typed sentences. Information on text readers is in Chapter 12, "Treatment and Technology to Improve Reading Comprehension."

- Be sure to connect this client and her family with associations, online discussion groups, and local support groups that are related to Parkinson's Disease. These are discussed in Chapter 19, "Online Support, Information, and Discussion Groups."

Scenario 5: Dealing With ALS

> A man with advanced ALS needs help communicating.

Technology Tips

- Take a look at Chapter 10, "Additional Tools and Resources To Improve Verbal Expression." It is likely that this person may benefit from a dedicated communication device. Many considerations are necessary to select the most appropriate one. Be sure that there are features that will help, as this person will require more assistance as this disease advances.

- Take a look at software such as EZ Keys by Words+ to minimize keystrokes while typing.

- Be sure to connect this person with ALS associations, online discussion groups, and local support groups that is discussed in Chapter 19, "Online Support, Information and Discussion Groups."

Scenario 6: Dealing With a Ruptured Aneurysm

> A patient is seen in the hospital several days after an aneurysm burst and is barely able to communicate.

Technology Tips

- Establish basic communication with the help of simple communication items such as The Vidatak E-Z board by Vidatak or the Critical Communicator by Interactive Therapeutics. There are also simple communication devices with voice such as the Go Talk by Attainment Company and Listen to Me by DTK Enterprises. These are reviewed in chapter 10, "Additional Tools and Resources To Improve Verbal Expression."

- Print out a personalized communication book with relevant information and pictures. This may be done quickly using therasimplicity.com's online subscription.

- Work closely with family to teach them how to communicate most effectively with environmental support such as pictures, maps, calendars and objects in view. Communication techniques may be printed from Web sites such as www.aphasia.org.

- Talk to family about ways to stimulate conversation, and how they can interact and engage the patient in stimulating activities, such as playing card games, looking at talking photo albums and talking about daily events and basic needs. These suggestions are reviewed at the beginning of Chapter 14, "Treatment and Technology To Improve Cognition and Memory."

- Be sure to review online resources and the ways technology and software might be able to help once the client is out of the acute care phase and into rehabilitation.

- Refer to the Acute Care setting section of Chapter 3, "Treatment Settings."

Scenario 7: Dealing With Speech Problems

A person is about to lose his job because others have trouble understanding his speech.

Technology Tips

- Establish speech patterns that more intelligible with the help of software designed for accent reduction. Examples include HearSay for All by Communication Disorders Technology, American Speech Sounds by Speech Com, and Pronunciation Power by English Learning. It is also helpful to use Sights and Sounds by Bungalow Software—especially the final lesson into which personalized text can be typed and voice recorded. These resources are reviewed in Chapter 9 "Treatment and Technology to Improve Verbal Expression."

- Print out lists from therasimplicity.com for speech practice or some of the free online resources to print listed in Chapter 16, "Multi-Media Programs and Generating Printed Treatment Materials." A particularly helpful site might be Caroline Bowden's lists of minimal pairs and listening lists for articulation and phonological therapy at ttp://members.tripod.com/CarolineBowen/wordlists.html.

- Explore sites listed in Chapter 17, "Games and Free Online Interactive Activities," such as www.englishclub.com, http://a4esl.org, and www.englishforum.com/00/interactive.

- Search for community-based groups in which to practice conversational skills. Try searching under "Google" and type in key words such as "ESL conversation groups" and the name of your city.

- Practice role-playing work-related situations with scripts and a video camera.

- Type work-related vocabulary and frequently used sentences into a word processing file and use text readers to practice saying the sentences aloud. Text readers are reviewed in the Assistive Reading Technology section of Chapter 12, "Treatment and Technology To Improve Reading Comprehension."

- Review the benefits of talking translators by companies such as those from Franklin Electronic Publishers. These resources are reviewed in Chapter 10, "Additional Tools and Resources To Improve Verbal Expression."

Scenario 8: Dealing With Apraxia of Speech

> A three-year-old boy with apraxia of speech is very frustrated because he can't make himself understood.

Technology Tips

- With a young child, therapy needs to be interactive and fun. It is helpful to play games and use a hands-on prompting technique for eliciting speech sounds.

- Helpful lists with which to work can be used from therasimplicity.com and other resources mentioned in Chapter 16, "Multi-Media Programs and Generating Printed Treatment Materials."

- Use pediatric games that can engage the child during the drill and practice tasks such as Bailey's Book House by The Learning Company or JumpStart Software by Knowledge Adventure. More gaming software can be found in Chapter 17, "Games and Free Online Interactive Activities."

- Use products that provide visual and graphic feedback of speech and voice production which are found in Chapter 9- "Treatment and Technology to Improve Verbal Expression." Examples include Dr. Speech and Sound Beginnings by Tool Time.

- If it is helpful to see up-close video of mouth movement as featured with the Speech Therapy CD by WinGo Global or Speech Sounds on Cue by Bungalow Software.

- The "It's a …" Bundle Therapy for Expressive Naming Disorders and Articulation I, II and II by Locutour are very helpful for repetition of targeted speech sounds.

Scenario 9: Dealing With Sports-related Injuries

> A 10th grader has had several sports-related injuries and his grades are falling in school.

Technology Tips

- Review organizational, memory and learning strategies the student uses. Suggestions and software to help with memory, organization, and thinking are reviewed in Chapter14, "Treatment and Technology To Improve Cognition and Memory." Encourage him to break down tasks into smaller steps.

- Make sure he has a good routine and environment for studying.

- If he needs help memorizing, try RecallPlus study software.

- Explore the benefits of using talking word processors with study tools, such as Read and Write Gold or Wynn Wizard to assist with reading, writing, and learning. These are reviewed in Chapter 12, "Treatment and Technology To Improve Reading Comprehension."

- To help with organization of written narrative, software that features outlining and webbing such as Inspiration by Inspiration Software may help. These are also discussed in Chapter 12.

- Encourage his family to participate in brain injury and learning disability related online discussion groups, and to review the sites of associations and organizations. This information is located in Chapter 19, "Online Support, Information, and Discussion Groups."

- Refer to the section on school in Chapter 3, "Treatment Settings" for additional treatment suggestions and helpful tools and strategies.

Scenario 10: Dealing With Language, Learning, and Literacy Challenges

A child in elementary school has difficulty participating in class due to poor English skills.

Technology Tips

- Use talking word processors such as IntelliTools and Clicker 5 to provide multi-sensory cues during literacy activities. These are discussed in Chapter 13, "Treatment and Technology To Improve Written Expression."

- Empower this child and the family to learn to use helpful technology for further practice of English both in school and at home. Start with Talk Now! English or World Talk English by EuroTalk. Other options are Rosetta Stone and Tell Me More English by Auralog, both of which offer online subscriptions. These resources are reviewed in Chapter 9, "Treatment and Technology To Improve Verbal Expression."

- Review electronic devices to help with translation, spelling, pronunciation, and language learning. English picture dictionaries are also helpful. These resources are reviewed in Chapter 10, "Additional Tools and Resources To Improve Verbal Expression."

- Show many of the free online interactive programs reviewed in Chapter 17, "Games and Free Online Interactive Activities." Examples include www.englishclub.com, http://a4esl.org and www.englishforum.com/00/interactive.

- Alternative book formats to support literacy may also help. These are discussed in the Alternative Book Formats section of Chapter 12, "Treatment and Technology To Improve Reading Comprehension. "

Chapter 5:
Software Selection

Technology can provide clients with a means to compensate for difficulties as well as to strengthen weak skills. It's important to keep in mind the goals and interests of the clients, as well as their ability to remember, learn, use their hands, and see the monitor. Because each person has unique desires, experiences, strengths, and limitations, a tool that is helpful in one situation or setting may be of little use in another. Selecting the appropriate technology requires a careful analysis of the interaction between the client, the task, the situation, and the software or other device.

The software and computer use in treatment should be selected so that they help the client reach established goals. However, if clients enjoy a computer-based activity, it doesn't necessarily mean that it is a waste of time for them to practice that activity on their own. There are many occasions when it is valuable to have clients engage in non-threatening and enjoyable activities. Many clients are dealing with new frustrations and significant changes in their lives and they need "down" time as much as we all do. A work/play balance is essential for all individuals; it should just not be confused with activities that are performed to help reach goals.

The information in this guide provides a broad range of guidance in the selection of tools that can be used to benefit a diverse group of people with a wide range of deficits in many settings. Some software titles are listed more than once in different categories and in different chapters to simplify the search process. All Web sites are provided. Please keep in mind that prices, specifications and Web sites change. Many products do offer demos and trials that are described online. An index of the software is provided at the end of this guide.

Treatment Goals

Treatment goals involving the use of technology can be grouped to accomplish a variety of tasks.

- Therapy can work toward learning to use resources to help compensate for areas of weakness. By compensating for certain abilities, the strategy practiced often improves the actual level of functioning.

- Therapy can be used to improve specific skills through drill and practice, with the hope of generating new neurological connections for those skills.

- Treatment can focus on generating a comprehensive independent practice program involving computer use, so that clients can practice on their own, outside of formal sessions.

- Treatment can include the exploration of resources which clients can use to enhance self-advocacy, overall quality of life and greater participation in social, work, school and leisure activities.

Ease of Use, Flexibility and Visual Presentation

Programs vary widely in the expertise required to achieve maximize benefit. Some are straightforward and intuitive, while others require advanced preparation and practice on the part of the clinician.

There are several strategies that clinicians can use to make the computer easier to use for clients:

- If one of the treatment goals is to have the client use the programs for independent practice, the programs should be easy to enter, exit, and resume.

- Directions should be clear and concise.

- Clinicians can help by placing shortcuts for programs on the desktop, writing a "tip sheet" for the client to remember specific ways to use programs, and providing simplified, step-by-step instructions for practicing suggested exercises.

- If a client does not have computer expertise and plans to practice programs outside of formal therapy sessions, a "computer buddy" is helpful. This designated person can help the client get started on the computer, load the software, and select the appropriate settings and options, along with other help as needed.

Clinicians may find the following guidelines helpful when learning to use new software:

- Learning to use software is most effective when watching an experienced clinician use the product with a client who has similar goals. Unfortunately, observing others is not often possible.

- Other options offered by some vendors are online tutorials and personal phone consultations to initiate the learning process. Chapter 19 lists many Web sites which provide tutorials and training for many AAC and AT products. They are listed under the section titled, "Sites Offering Assistive Technology Training and Information."

- Repeated exposure to and practice with software are needed to retain knowledge of the features in a program, the type of client for whom it is most appropriate, and which goals it most effectively addresses.

Think about the options provided by a program when deciding whether it is a good match for a client.

- Some software products, such as Talk Now! American English by EuroTalk, Speech Practice by Wingo Global, and CHAT (Computerized Home Aphasia Therapy) by Aphasia Therapy Products do not offer customizable preferences. They are what they are and can be appropriate selections if they are a good fit. They may be used differently with different people, but options cannot be selected.

- In contrast, Bungalow Software, Laureate Software, some of the Parrot Software, and advanced text readers with study support features offer quite a few choices, so that tasks are optimized for each person.

- Customizable choices may include features such as determining the number of items in a lesson, the type of cues and reinforcement, the speed at which the text is read aloud, and visual presentation of the stimulus.

Program flexibility should also be considered, not only in terms of its ability to adapt to the needs of an individual, but also with regard to how it may be applied to meet the needs of different types of clients in different situations.

- Software is more valuable in a school or rehabilitation setting if it can be used to work toward improving or compensating for a variety of skills and needs for multiple clients in a caseload.

- Each person has a unique personality, learning style, type of communication, and cognitive profile. It's up to the therapist to tap into the available resources in the best way possible to maximize the effectiveness of time spent in treatment and in home practice.

- Programs such as CHAT, Speech Therapy by Wingo Global, the Aphasia Tutor Series by Bungalow Software, Parrot Software by Parrot Software, Clicker 5 by Crick Software, and Dollars and Cents by Attainment Company use large text and graphics. These are ideal for people with visual or perceptual difficulties.

- Other programs, such as Moriarty Mystery by Bungalow Software, and Looking for Words by Attainment Company are visually complex and can be difficult to navigate for clients with visual impairments. However, clinicians may decide to use the more complex software such as Looking for Words to work on improving visual and perceptual skills. This can be done by having the client use strategies to find named items.

Computer Program Response and Feedback

The simplest programs offer stimuli a client can use for practice that don't require additional direct computer interaction. The clients sit, watch, and hopefully verbalize along with the program. Other programs provide drill and practice exercises that require typing, talking, or direct selection of items on the computer and then offer feedback regarding the accuracy of the user response.

The "load and use" programs that do not provide feedback

- do not involve customization,

- do not offer options,

- do not require much clicking or other direct computer interaction to move from one item to the next, and

- do not provide feedback regarding the accuracy of the response.

Examples of this type of program include World Talk English by EuroTalk and Speech Sounds on Cue by Bungalow Software.

The software programs that provide drill-and-practice tasks to improve targeted skills typically have the following characteristics:

- The therapist first configures the software, so that the client is working at the appropriate level of difficulty with the optimal feedback, stimuli, and number of trials.

- Once the user selects an item or provides input with the keyboard, mouse or microphone, feedback is provided regarding the accuracy of the response. Either the program automatically continues to the next item, or the user indicates, through a click of the mouse, his or her readiness to proceed.

- Intuitive programs use a natural progression of task difficulty.

Some of these programs include Dollars and Cents by Attainment Software, Language Learning Software by Rosetta Stone, and the Aphasia Tutor Series. Parrot Software offers an extensive variety of programs that are intuitive to use once the appropriate program has been selected. Many offer multiple lessons that progressively become more challenging.

Clicker 5, the Lingraphica by Lingraphicare, and Universal Reader by Premiere Assistive Technology are examples of programs that are relatively easy for the client or student to use, but require knowledge on the part of the therapist to set them up correctly.

Customization of Software Content

A useful feature of some software is authoring capability, which is the ability to customize the content of the stimuli. Such programs enable the therapist to select pictures, input text, and record voice for a particular individual. Programs such as Clicker 5 and ClozePro by Crick Software, and some of the Bungalow Software such as Sights 'n Sounds, enable the therapist to provide the stimulus items. Names of family members, interesting newspaper articles, and digital pictures of a person's house may be used in these programs for increased interest.

Time Requirement

Keep in mind how much time the software will be used during a given session. Certain programs lend themselves to short treatment times. Others, such as Memory Works' A Day in a Life by The Practical Memory Institute or Moriarty Mystery, require more time to complete.

Use of Traditional Therapy

Computer use is not always the most effective way to deliver rehabilitation and literacy intervention services. If accessing a computer is time-consuming, the computer isn't functioning properly, or the client is not be able to practice between sessions, other treatment techniques may be more appropriate. In the acute care setting, a good use of time might include providing the client a list of computer and Internet resources to pursue after discharge, as treatment time is so limited. In the home, if family members are not comfortable with computers or a computer is difficult to access, workbooks and other items might be more worthwhile.

Number of Stimuli Items and Order of Presentation

Many programs have hundreds of items to practice; others have only a few. Certain software allows the user to select either automatic randomization of items or consistent presentation of items. Some programs enable the user to select different lessons of either the same level of difficulty or differing levels and to choose the number of items in a lesson.

Language and Cognitive Tasks Required in the Program

It's important to dissect the task at hand to ascertain what language and cognitive skills are required to use a program and what goals are addressed during use of the program. The cognitive abilities of attention, concentration, sequencing, reasoning, and memory are integral to performing many computer activities. Language is also involved in many tasks in the form of reading, writing, talking, or listening. Some software has been developed specifically for practicing language and cognitive skills. Other software requires the user to have many of these skills already in order to practice skills that are more complex.

Cost

There is considerable variation in the cost of products. Many products can be purchased in more than one location and may be priced differently depending on the place of purchase. Some software can be downloaded at no expense, while other tools and devices cost thousands of dollars. In this guide, Web sites are listed for resources described. The sites give prices for individual products. Please keep in mind that prices frequently change and that software can be repackaged with other products. Many programs are available in professional or consumer versions, may have network versions, and may have package prices for multiple copies or use on more than one computer.

When establishing a budget for using computers in speech therapy, it is necessary to consider the additional hidden costs of software use. For example, there may be expenses to pay someone to install the software, train the user, maintain the computers, and purchase updates as they are developed.

Context and Situation

Keep in mind the context in which the software will be used. Clinicians work in a wide variety of settings. Some will continue to provide support to clients as they use the suggested software, while others will discharge clients after the recommendations are made. Work settings where therapy is provided include acute care hospitals, rehabilitation hospitals, long-term care settings, regular and specialized education settings, work and community re-entry programs, outpatient clinics, clients' homes, and private practices. Possible scenarios include the user practicing assignments at home, at school, or at work and using the software in social and recreational situations. The environment and the purpose for use of software or a device are of paramount importance. Technology may compensate for a problem in one setting, but be ineffective in another. The user may be distracted by extraneous noise, have inadequate support, or cause problems if the talking programs are disturbing to others. Social Networks is a tool to use during the evaluation process to identify important variables affecting communication and to guide interventions that may affect the development of communication skills over time. Social Networks is a product that takes a "person centered" approach to developing AAC strategies, actively involving the individual along with those people most likely to be knowledgeable about his or her communication behaviors. More information can be found at www.augcominc.com.

Program Format: Internet, CD or Fully Loaded

Resources such as the online versions by Parrot Software, Rosetta Stone, TheraSimplicity by Simplicity Software, News-2-You Online Newspaper by News-2-You, NeuroPsychOnline by Psychological Software Services, and Tell Me More by Auralog require access to the Internet. Other software programs, such as Looking for Words and Speech Sounds on Cue require a CD. Some products are available in either format, such as software by Rosetta Stone and Pronunciation Power by English Computerized Learning. There are also products by Bungalow Software, WordQ2 by Quillsoft and Speech Practice that can be loaded onto the computer's hard drive, eliminating the need for the CD. The format for the software is important when the physical location for computer use is established.

Clarity of Directions and Phone Support

Programs developed specifically for helping people with disabilities tend to have the most helpful phone support. Parrot Software, Bungalow Software, and Premier Assistive Technologies consistently provide timely and helpful phone assistance. Several of the companies that produce high-end products, such as Kurzweil Educational Systems, DynaVox Systems, and Prentke Romich Company, often have representatives who may be available to offer onsite support.

Programs developed for professionals who help people with communication and cognitive challenges most often come with written documentation, online information, or directions that can be accessed on the computer once the program is loaded. Bungalow Software, Laureate Software, Parrot Software, Crick Software, NeuroPsychOnline, Premiere Assistive Technology, and Rosetta Stone are supported with helpful documentation. Products produced primarily for teaching English as a second language, for helping people with low vision use a computer, or to help with business productivity can be helpful speech therapy tools, but do not come with written suggestions of how to use them in therapy. It's up to the resourceful clinician to use those tools successfully.

Recording Data

It's beneficial for both the client and the therapist to use software programs that record responses and document progress. Often, clients might feel discouraged and have difficulty believing that gains are being made. Written evidence can help them realize that the treatment and their hard work are making a difference. Recorded performance data assists the therapist in adapting programs as needed to achieve the desired outcome. Such data can also document the need for more intervention. Reviewing the results of practice sessions is also helpful when analyzing home practice assignments.

Chapter 6:
Computer Access, Customization, and Hardware Selection

Computers can provide a new world of independence for people with physical, communication, or cognitive disabilities. Designing environments, products, and information to be easily used by the greatest number of people, with or without disabilities — has become much more prevalent in the development of technological products. This translates into mainstream technology that is more accessible and that serves the different needs and personal preferences of many users, including people with communication and cognitive deficits. Many hardware options and mainstream products can now be modified to provide functional and more affordable alternatives for users with disabilities.

Computer hardware can be configured to do the following tasks:

- Provide alternate direct selection modes for people who can't use an everyday keyboard and mouse.
- Help manage organization and memory tasks.
- Activate environmental controls such as turning on the lights or selecting a television channel.
- Speak for people who are unable to talk, via dedicated communication devices and screen readers.
- Read aloud written material for people who can understand what is said, but not what is written.

For clinicians, administrators, clients, and families who may not be well versed in computer use, it can be an overwhelming experience to select, purchase, and configure the appropriate hardware to accommodate for disabilities. The following is a brief introduction to some of the options available, including suggestions about where to begin when purchasing computers and peripherals for use in therapy.

Computer Access

One of the first steps when working with a client is to determine which method of computer access is the most appropriate. During the initial assessment, it is preferable to have access to a variety of monitors, keyboards, and direct selection devices. When a client has multiple physical issues and may benefit from help with positioning, adapted switches, or other complex access issue, a multi-disciplinary assistive technology team is ideal to establish the best method of computer access. Once the client has the appropriate setup, the clinician providing the communication and cognitive treatment can then continue to work with the individual on developing a strategy for the use of technology to improve and compensate for communication, cognitive, literacy and community-based challenges.

Here are two products on the market that might help with this process. Additional suggestions are described in Chapter 2, "Getting Started."

COMPASS
by Koester Performance Research (KRP), www.kpronline.com

- Compass software measures the user's skills during computer interactions.

- It is designed to help clinical and educational professionals perform computer access evaluations with their clients and students. Skills assessed include keyboard and mouse use, navigation through menus, and switch use.

- It includes eight skill tests, covering text entry, and the use of pointing devices and switches.

- Each test has many configuration options to customize testing as needed. Compass collects speed and accuracy data during test performance and reports the results.

- Windows

- $179.00

EvaluWare
by AssistiveWare, www.assistiveware.com

- EvaluWare is a software program that was developed to identify the best computer access methods and ideal AAC (Augmentative and Alternative Communication) setups for users with special needs.

- It combines several types of assessments into one package to identify the best settings and preferences for the user based on motor/access, looking, listening and other related skills.

- Motor and access skills are assessed through identifying the learner's appropriate input method and settings using a touch screen, mouse, switch, keyboard, or alternative pointer.

- Visual skills are assessed through identifying the learner's ideal visual target size, number of items, and type of image.

- Listening skills are assessed through identifying the learner's preferred voice, and type of feedback.

- This program assess the readiness of the user to use an on-screen keyboard and word prediction software.
- Windows and Mac
- $125.00

Single Switch Software

Some individuals with significant motoric impairments need obtain access to the computer with the use of switches and scanning. The process of scanning involves many skills such as controlling the switch, attending to the auditory and visual stimuli on the computer monitor, and the discrimination of the visual symbols and auditory feedback. It is also important to keep in mind the optimal body positioning, location, and mounting of the switch and type of switch to be used.

For more information, please refer to www.geocities.com/learntoscan for an article by Robert Koch in *Closing the Gap* in December of 2006 and for a free software guide for beginner scanners.

When a client is only able to access software via a single switch, software selection is more limited. Many of the products described in this guide are accessible for people who need to use a switch. More detailed guidance on the use of technology for these users can be found at the following two Web sites.

- www.switchintime.com — This Web site by the developers of Scan 'n Read has quite a few free programs for the Macintosh platform. Downloads include CD Jukebox, Single Switch Bingo, Scan 'n Read, and Word Search.
- www.judylynn.com — Judy Lynn produces a variety of switch software for people with special needs.

Computer Specifications and Operating System

Old vs. New Computer

As time passes, computers improve and costs decrease. Clients frequently inquire about the advantages and disadvantages of using a computer they may already own, or purchasing a new one. It isn't necessary to purchase the newest and most expensive computers for education and rehabilitation in order to benefit from assistive technology and multimedia programs to improve communication, cognition, and literacy. Most computers purchased within the past five years should be sufficient for therapy use if there is enough free space on the hard drive. Even the least expensive new computers are more than adequate and may actually be better than products available just a year or two ago. However, new complex software products with voice recognition or extensive graphics do sometimes require significant amounts of memory and often function better with higher-speed computers. Specific computer requirements for particular software products are listed on their Web sites. All computers should be equipped with a CD-ROM or DVD player, speakers, microphone, and sound card.

It can be helpful to consult with computer-savvy friends and colleagues when purchasing a new computer. Computer magazine reviews, such as *PC Magazine* at www.pcmag.com and *Consumer Reports* at www.consumerreports.com, are often also insightful.

Computer-Operating Platforms: Mac, Windows and Open Source

Most specialized software that was produced for rehabilitation and education was initially produced for the Macintosh (Mac) computer. Times changed, and it appears that Microsoft took the lead and became the mainstream product in most places. Macintosh computers are once again becoming increasingly popular due to their ease of use. There are also "open source" platforms such as Linux. These platforms are available for anyone to use, modify, and redistribute freely.

The vast majority of schools, rehabilitation centers, and individuals are most familiar with the Microsoft-based personal computers (PCs). However, if a client already owns a Mac, software by Microsoft called Virtual PC, available at www.microsoft.com, will enable a Mac to use PC-only software. Some Macs have divided platforms for both Mac and PC. Quite a bit of software is also hybrid and can be used with either platform.

With all of these systems, users can adjust screen colors, contrast, resolution, text and icon size, visual sound alerts, cursor size, and cursor speed. Their operating systems also include onscreen keyboard, screen reader, text-to-speech, and magnifier programs. Instructions are generally located within the operating systems "help menu." Web site information is listed in this guide as products are reviewed. The sites specify the platforms their products are compatible with and the software and hardware requirements.

Macintosh Computers

Macintosh computers offer built-in accessibility features such as VoiceOver, QuickTime, Text Track, Speech Recognition, Text-to-Speech Synthesis, and other tools that can be adapted to meet the unique needs of each learner. Apple refers to these features collectively as Universal Access. More information can be found at www.apple.com/education/accessibilitysolution. The operating system is scheduled to change in mid-2007 from the Tiger operating system to the Leopard operating system. The accessibility options in this new operating system are said to be more advanced than with the current system.

Personal Computers

Windows XP has most recently been the standard Microsoft platform. Details and tutorials about its accessibility options can be found at the Web site www.microsoft.com/enable.

A new Windows operating system called Vista was released in early 2007. There are some known compatibility issues with software and the author of this guide has not used the software in this guide with Vista. Vista includes built-in accessibility settings and programs that make it easier for computer users to see, hear, and use their computers. The accessibility settings and programs in Windows Vista are helpful to people with visual difficulties, hearing loss, pain in their hands or arms, or reasoning and cognitive issues. More information can be found at www.microsoft.com.

Computer Format — Desktops, Notebooks, Tablets, Handhelds, and Portable Word Processors

Computers are available in a wide variety of formats, including desktops, laptops or notebooks, tablets, handhelds, and portable word processors. Each type of computer has pros and cons. Some computers now are available with integrated touch screens, wireless Internet access, and the capacity to accommodate adapted keyboards and other alternate input devices.

During the selection process, it is necessary to consider

- the degree of mobility needed,
- compatibility with other computers the client may be using,
- the cost, and
- the location of electrical outlets, wiring and lighting.

Desktops

Desktop computers are the easiest to use for most individuals and often provide the greatest value for equivalent specifications. They have standard keyboards and large monitors and can easily be set up with accommodations for people with physical limitations. Desktops are typically used when there is one designated computer location. Unless they are located on moving workstations, they are difficult to transport.

Notebooks/Laptops

Notebook computers have almost all the functionality of regular desktop computers. In recent years, the price gap has narrowed considerably with equivalent desktop computers. Compared to a desktop alternative, they are easier to transport and store. However, when compared to tablets and handheld devices, their weight prevents them from being easily transported. They have longer initial startup times when compared to those of dedicated communication devices. The keyboards are smaller than those of desktops, and may be difficult to use for people who have visual or manual dexterity issues.

- Accommodations can make notebook computers easier to use. Regular keyboards can be attached, alternate mice and trackballs can be used, and talking software can read aloud text shown on the monitor.

- An advantage of this type of computer over a desktop computer in education and rehabilitation is that it can be used during treatment sessions and then brought home for practice. Clinicians can also transport theirs to a client's home or other setting.

- Many people actively debate between getting a notebook to be used for communication or a dedicated communication device that is used exclusively to augment verbal expression. It may be less costly to add communication software to a notebook and the notebook computer can be used with other applications. On the downside, notebooks typically have a shorter battery life, are bulkier, and require a longer amount of time to "boot up" than a dedicated device.

- There is also much debate in the schools whether students who would benefit from assistive technology to help with reading and writing should use a notebook computer or a portable word processor such as the Dana by Alphasmart. Laptops are great because they enable the user to use additional software, and access the Internet. They may also use software that is similar to the software used on desktop computers. Portable word processors are easy to carry and are less expensive.

- Some manufacturers, such as Panasonic, produce "rugged" computers with touch screens that hold up well in adverse conditions for computers. One example is the Panasonic Toughbook Series at www.panasonic.com/toughbook.

Tablet Computers

Table computers look like the screen of a laptop. They typically run a different version of XP called XP Tablet. However, with the new smaller models of tablets, there are "big Windows" applications on a small Windows XP Pro-based computer.

- Instead of a keyboard, a tablet pen or the voice is used to navigate and add data directly onto the screen.

- It can be docked to a station in order to use a keyboard, CD/DVD drive, or other peripherals if desired.

- Tablet computers are easily transported compared to notebook computers, but are heavier than portable word processors and handhelds.

- Many tablet computers now offer the ability to convert handwriting into editable text. However, as with voice recognition, this may require significant training time with the computer until it learns the user's handwriting.

- Tools are now available for speech recognition, magnification, and screen reading.

- Less software is available for most tablets than for desktops or notebooks, and they are generally more expensive than desktop computers.

- A commercial comparison site for further information can be found at www.tabletpc2.com/Compare.htm.

Handhelds

Handhelds are also referred to as personal digital assistants (PDAs), Palms, and Pocket PCs. They are becoming increasingly popular for business, personal use, education, and rehabilitation. There are many products coming on the market that fall in this category that offer many benefits such as the following:

- They can be used to help with organization, data entry, task management, and augmentative communication.

- Due to their small size, handhelds are great if used as a communication device or as a help with memory.

- Many types are now available in telephones that are combined with pocket PCs or Palm operating systems. They are referred to as "smart phones." Because they are light and small, these devices are extremely mobile.

- They feature an "instant on," so lengthy boot times are not needed.

- Depending on the model and how the device is used, at least one day of operation is typically available on a battery charge.

- Many accessories and applications are becoming increasingly available and are useful when clients have intact vision and fine motor control. Accessories such as portable full-size keyboards and text readers are available to make them easier to use.

- Handhelds can be synched to a larger computer on which it is easier to enter data.

- Infrared beaming allows the transfer of data without cables or external services, and wireless Internet access is now available on most models.

Despite these benefits, PDAs are currently not appropriate for all users. There are several drawbacks:

- Good fine motor control and vision are needed.

- The devices can be easily misplaced.

- The small screen is difficult on the eyes when used for sustained viewing.

- They are not appropriate for people who cannot use the stylus or see the screen.

- A growing number of assistive technologies are available for PDAs, but those technologies are often developed for only one of the major operating systems (Palm OS or Microsoft Pocket PC), not both.

- Due to limitations of memory and processing power, most PDA applications tend to have fewer accessibility options compared to desktop computers.

- Speech recognition, text-to-speech, augmentative communication, and graphic organization software has recently entered the market and may increase the usability of these devices for people with disabilities.

Additional information is available at the accessibility pages for the leading PDA operating system vendors:

- PalmOne Accessibility Program: http://www.palm.com/us/company/corporate/pap

- Microsoft Accessibility: www.microsoft.com/enable/

For more information about the use of handhelds to help people with communication and cognitive deficits refer to the Chapter 14, "Treatment and Technology To Improve Cognition and Memory." Also, check out these Web sites:

- www.ablelink.com

- www.handango.com

- www.inspiration.com

- www.gusinc.com

- www.readingmadeeasy.com

- www.brainaid.com

- www.assistivetech.com

Portable Word Processors

Portable word processors combine the affordability of a handheld with the ergonomic benefits of a notebook computer. They also provide a long battery life that allows days of typical use on a single charge. Portable word processors are used to do the following tasks:

- Record notes

- Use a calculator

- Improve readability of text

- Organize priorities with to-do lists

- Select directly with a touch screen

- Read and write e-mail

- Browse the Internet

- Access Palm- or PC-based software

Cursors

Cursors can be very difficult for people with visual perceptual deficits to find and use. There are several options available for enlarging the size of the cursor:

- To access options on a computer with a Windows operating system, click Start, click Control Panel, double click on the Mouse icon, and click on the Pointer tab on the properties page. Below "Scheme" is a drop-down box that contains predefined sets of mouse pointers you can use. Click on this box and pick one of the large, extra large, or inverted schemes.

- You can also make the mouse pointer more visible by adding pointer trails, on the Pointer Options page

- For more highly visible mouse pointers, free downloads are available at http://www.gusinc.com/bigcursor.html. The downloads can be put into a folder and accessed from the mouse pointer "scheme" browse button.

Selection Devices

The standard mouse may be fine for most people with good hand control. However, many people with disabilities have impaired fine motor movements and find it difficult to see the movement of the cursor on the computer screen. Some people are unable to use their dominant hand due to weakness, paralysis, or coordination deficits. It takes practice to use the mouse with the non-preferred hand. Fortunately, a wide variety of mice and trackballs are on the market.

Trackballs are often good solutions because the cursor can be controlled with a finger. The device stays in one place as the user moves the ball. There are quite a few trackballs available at many computer stores. The BIGtrack is the largest trackball available. The large ball requires less fine motor control than a standard trackball, and it is ruggedly built.

Technology is also available to assist people with little or no use of their hands. People who have reliable movement of just about any part of their body can control the cursor on the screen. Reliable mouth movement or even eye gaze can control the computer. Special switches make use of at least one muscle over which the individual has voluntary control, such as the head, knee, or mouth. To make selections, clients use switches activated by movement. The wireless IntelliSwitch by IntelliTools at www.intellitools.com, engineered by Madentec, provides wireless access to most switch accessible software. People who have severe mobility impairments often can use scanning and Morse code for computer access. People who have very low vision/blindness can use tactile systems such as Braille for computer access. Vendors specializing in Technology for the blind can be found at the Web sites www.nyise.org/vendors.htm and www.visiontech.svrc.vic.edu.au/brailleaccess.htm.

Monitors

A large, flat-panel, LCD (liquid crystal display) monitor is preferable for the clear image and space-saving features over the CRT (cathode ray tube) alternative that is much bulkier.

If the computer user has difficulty using a mouse or a trackball, a touch screen may be an appropriate solution. Touch screens can be attached or integrated into the monitor itself. Integrated touch screens are more reliable, but expensive. The touch screens that attach to monitors are more affordable, but are more likely to lose their calibration and break down. Sometimes touch screens complicate the issue; clients may inadvertently touch the screen when they don't intend to select an item. Various prices and types are available. Further information is available at www.enablemart.com and www.mayer-johnson.com.

Keyboards

Whenever possible, clinicians should use mainstream products such as a standard keyboard with clients.

Keyguards and keyboard overlays are helpful accessories when needed. They can

- decrease the number of unwanted keystrokes due to someone with poor manual coordination hitting more than one key at a time,

- keep the mechanics of a keyboard safe from the effects of spills and drooling, and

- help individuals identify the keys.

Several adapted keyboards used frequently are Intellikeys and Big Keys LX.

IntelliKeys USB
by Intellitools of Cambian Learning, www.intellitools.com

- IntelliKeys USB plugs into the computer's USB port and provides access for people with physical, visual, or cognitive disabilities who have difficulty using a standard keyboard.

- Unlike the standard keyboard, the visual presentation and function can be customized by sliding in different overlays.

- IntelliKeys comes with six standard overlays that are ready to use with any word processing program or software that has keyboard input. Windows or Mac compatible. $395.00

Big Keys Plus
by Greystone Digital Inc., www.bigkeys.com and available at www.infogrip.com

- This is a standard size keyboard with 1-inch keys. There is a multi-colored, QWERTY key layout.

Windows XP includes special features that can help with keyboard use. To access those features, go to Programs, Accessories, and then Accessibility Options, or find the Accessibilities Options folder in the Control Panel.

Expanded keyboards that have larger keys spaced farther apart can replace standard keyboards for people with limited fine motor control. Mini-keyboards provide access for those who have fine motor control, but lack the range of motion to use a standard keyboard. There are also keyboard trays with adjustable arms can be purchased for individualized positioning of the client.

Speech and Voice Input

Speech input provides another option for people with disabilities who have difficulty typing. Through voice-recognition technology, the user controls the computer by speaking into a microphone. A particular system is trained to recognize specific voices. These products are very difficult for clients to use who have communication and cognitive deficits. There is a new product called SpeakQ by Quillsoft (www.wordq.com) that was produced to help people with disabilities benefit from voice recognition technology.

Voice input can also be used for environmental control with environmental control units (ECUs.) Commands can be given for turning lights on and off, adjusting room temperature, and operating appliances when coupled with an environmental control unit or program. For more information about this type of technology, check out www.abilityhub.com/speech/speech-ecu.htm.

Headsets and Microphone

Much of the software described in this guide is for recording and listening to speech. It is often a sound investment to purchase a good set of headphones with a built-in microphone for use with voice recording and voice recognition software. External noise reduction features are helpful. If a client and clinician are working in a noisy environment or if the speech of the computer will disturb others, headphones with a splitter are helpful so that both people can hear the computer. Good quality headphones with microphones can be found in most computer supply stores that sell voice recognition software.

If the user uses a hearing aid or is not comfortable with a headset, a desktop microphone can be purchased. These are readily available at computer stores and Radio Shack.

Networks

- The main benefit of a network is that it allows more than one computer to share resources such as Internet connections, storage space, printers, and applications.

- Remote access enables people to access a computer from different locations.

- Networks facilitate group collaboration, allowing the sharing of calendars, files and even simultaneous sharing of applications.

- A downside to the use of networks is that they add a level of complexity and outside help will typically be needed to install, configure, and maintain them.

- Quite a bit of the software described in this guide is available in a network version. Specific information about the networking versions and pricing can be found on the Web sites listed for each product.

Protection

Safeguards need to be in place to protect the computer and the personal information stored on it.

- Quality surge protectors are needed to avoid harm from thunderstorms and other electrical surges.

- Virus, spyware, and firewall protection keep the computer free of harmful external influences.

- Frequent software updates keep things running smoothly.

- Passwords to prevent unauthorized access should be used.

Additional Resources

More detailed information and guidance about the selection and purchase of hardware is offered on the following Web sites:

- Ability Hub, www.abilityhub.com

- Apple Accessibility, www.apple.com/accessibility

- AssistiveTech.net, www.assistivetech.net

- Assistive Technology Center, www.atechcenter.net

- Microsoft Accessibility, www.microsoft.com/enable

- Madentec, www.madentec.com

- RehabTool.com, www.rehabtool.com

Chapter 7:
Computer Setup Considerations

Professionals help people with communication and cognition challenges in a wide variety of settings with many different types of patients, clients, and students. Each scenario requires different computer setup considerations and solutions. Some settings are quiet, while others have many distractions. Some settings have many restrictions for loading software, while others are limitless. Some settings have networked computers, while others have stand-alone workstations.

Here are some considerations to keep in mind when forming or expanding computer use in the treatment process:

- Type of setting such as a hospital, school or private office
- Multiple computers in a lab vs. stand-alone system
- Internet and networking availability
- Software storage
- Nature of goals most frequently addressed
- Software installation protocols
- Training and computer expertise of clients, professionals, and other support people
- Available funding and gradual vs. one-time approach toward acquisition of materials

One Computer in a Quiet Location

The use of one computer in a quiet location is the simplest situation to set up.

- Networking is not an issue.
- Individual programs can be purchased.
- Distractions are minimal.
- Practice with verbal expression tasks will not disturb others.

Several Treatment Rooms With One Computer in Each Location

When several treatment rooms each have one computer, the setup is a bit more involved. Considerations should include:

- The need to purchase multiple copies of software or devices

- Easy access of software by more than one clinician

- Potential restrictions regarding installation of new software or the ability to download from the Internet

- Logistics for networking common peripherals and online access.

More Than One Computer in a Large Room Setup for Independent Practice

The use of multiple computers in one room is often used so that people can independently practice between formal treatment sessions.

Clients often are set up in a lab with folders containing specific practice suggestions and assignments. It is generally helpful to have certain computers designated for different uses. For example, one computer could be for clients who need a touch screen and a large keyboard. Software could be loaded on that computer that is geared toward clients with communication and cognitive deficits and physical limitations that are more significant. Another computer could be loaded with high-level cognitive software. There are clients who need to use a touch screen that may be working on higher-level programs, but targeting types of clients for certain computers should enable the clinician to get more mileage out of the software and minimize the number of duplicate copies. It may be advisable to have clients focus on reading, writing, auditory comprehension, and cognitive tasks rather than verbal expression when in a lab with other clients or students, so that they don't disturb others.

Considerations for this scenario include:

- The level of support needed for people using the computer for independent practice

- The ability to customize a computer for particular client needs

- The method of access for the client to the appropriate lessons and configurations for practice

- Documentation procedures for practice and progress

- Ways to limit distractions when others are in the room, for example, by type of software and use of headphones

Internet Access

The use of the Internet is highly recommended during treatment sessions. It can be used to work on all aspects of communication and cognition and to generate therapy materials. More and more treatment solutions are offered online.

The use of Internet access is discussed in many chapters of this guide. Chapters 16 and 18 discuss many online resources that can be used to enhance treatment as well as free interactive sites that provide help with word retrieval, graphics, online games and activities, and disability-related support and information. There are also subscription-based programs such as Parrot, Rosetta Stone, and Tell Me More that are helpful for drill and practice of communication skills which are discussed in Chapter 8- "Treatment and Technology to Improve Verbal Expression." Chapter 17 discusses helpful Internet Communication Tools. Chapter 14 talks about adapted email, search engines and Web browsers and Chapter 15 reviews sites for free treatment materials, sources for pictures and online programs for generating treatment material.

Networking

It is a sound investment to network computers. There are wired and wireless options. In lab settings, networks can reduce licensing costs by making software available to multiple computers. Each computer gains access to the Internet, and peripherals such as printers and scanners are shared. Network compatibility options for the software discussed in this guide are documented on the product Web sites.

Software Storage

It's important to establish a system for software storage and easy access to software when there are multiple treatment rooms. When several clinicians are using the software and computers, it's preferable to have a centralized location with easy access to materials, and a sign-out and reservation system for the software. A filing system can be used to organize the software either alphabetically or by treatment modality. An effective system is to organize the software in alphabetical order and cross-reference it by treatment goal. For instance, in the "Reading" folder, the text-reading software and software companies such as Universal Reader, Kurzweil, Merit, Lexia, and ReadPlease can be listed. The actual programs and their specific instructions, as well as their license numbers and manuals, are in alphabetical order. "Quick Tips" can be placed in each file for reference by the clinician about things to remember while using the software. CDs are stored in protective sleeves and CD binders. Boxes are discarded to save space.

Nature of Goals Most Frequently Addressed

An initial investment should be concentrated on software that will be the most flexible in helping clients reach the goals most frequently addressed in therapy. This guide presents suggestions for these purchases in two ways. Chapters 8-13 present software for particular treatment goals including verbal expression, auditory comprehension, reading comprehension, written expression and cognition and memory. Chapter 2 focuses on software that is helpful to meet the needs of clinicians in particular work settings such as hospitals and schools. Chapter 3 presents scenarios of how to get started with clients with a specific diagnosis.

Software Installation

The installation of new software programs should be a gradual process. Be sure to close programs that are open before you install something new. Reboot the computer after loading each program. Too many programs loaded at once can cause a computer to slow down or crash. Certain programs may be incompatible, and the only way to know which program caused a glitch is to add them individually and use the computer after each one to make sure things are functioning properly.

Training and Computer Expertise of Clients, Professionals, and Other Support People

After learning about the features and intricacies of the software and devices, the next step is to devise a system to ensure that the hardware and software are used effectively. As the number of software programs increases, use this guide to help review software choices for particular goal areas. Clinicians often become accustomed to using particular software in certain ways and forget about other software and the many options available for meeting different client needs.

It is helpful to work closely with each client's support network. This may include professionals, family members, friends, and "computer buddies." Before discharge, everyone should be comfortable with the implementation of recommendations in the computer-based, individualized practice program.

Chapter 8:
Supportive Research

As software and assistive devices become more available and affordable, clinicians need to be aware of evidence-based, treatment practice and efficacy studies to ensure the highest quality of care possible. Increasingly, people are asking to see the "evidence" on which theories, practices, and products are based. There is a need for research and outcome studies to document the impact of assistive technology both to compensate for and to improve communication and cognitive skills in the fields of education and rehabilitation. People need to be convinced that the use of technology is helpful and is not merely a crutch that will hold people back.

The research literature is a valuable resource for evaluating the usefulness of technology in treatment and the ideal conditions for the treatment. Fortunately, a collection of clinical and medical evidence is slowly building to show that therapeutic intervention with the use of technology and computers can improve communication and cognition. As mentioned throughout this guide, it's critical that the needs and abilities of each client be matched with appropriate technological resources and used in a way to achieve the greatest results. This requires considerable professional experience and expertise.

It is important to keep in mind, that studies often do not address the wide array of people with communication and cognitive deficits seen for therapy or target the specific skill addressed in a treatment program. Technology is changing so fast that it's difficult for research to keep up with it. The research results, therefore, are often not applicable to the use of the latest technologies that might be most helpful for our clients. In addition, it's important to keep in mind that the effectiveness of technology to maximize treatment results depends on how the technology is implemented.

The suggested treatment approaches and use of resources described in this guide are based on the following three concepts:

Brain Neuroplasticity

Because of their neuroplastic qualities, brains are able to change and recover when given appropriate stimulation. Growing evidence suggests that lifestyle factors and cognitively challenging activities might help ward off or delay the onset of neurodegenerative diseases, possibly by building connections between brain cells or even spurring the production of new brain cells.

Treatment Intensity

In appropriate candidates, the intensity of treatment provided directly correlates to the rate and extent of progress made. Clients can practice for hours a day on the computer and therefore increase their treatment intensity. Brain-fitness exercises have been shown to help prevent or delay cognitive decline.

Compensation and Multimedia Treatment

The use of compensatory strategies and multimedia treatment can often improve the communication or cognitive impairment.

Research and Efficacy Studies

It is beyond the scope of this guide to provide a thorough review of current research results. However, for those who would like to review the available literature, here are some helpful leads.

American Heart Association Stroke Journal, http://stroke.ahajournals.org
This site reviews many clinical research trials related to stroke. One of particular interest is "Intensity of Aphasia Therapy, Impact on Recovery" at the following Web site: http://stroke.ahajournals.org/cgi/content/abstract/34/4/987.

Apraxia-Kids, www.apraxia-kids.org
This site offers a section on research at the following Web site: www.apraxia-kids.org/site/c.chKMI0PIIsE/b.788461/k.6CED/Apraxia_Research_Index/apps/nl/newsletter3.asp. A few studies talk about the need for intensive therapy for both children and adults with apraxia in order to maximize progress.

American Speech-Language Hearing Association (ASHA), www.asha.org
ASHA provides a searchable database of research studies.

Augmentative and Alternative Communication Rehabilitation Engineering Research Centers (AAC-RERC), www.aac-rerc.com
The AAC-RERC conducts a comprehensive program of research, development, training, and dissemination activities that address the National Institute on Disability and Rehabilitation Research (NIDRR) NIDRR priorities and seeks to improve technologies for individuals who rely on augmentative and alternative communication (AAC) technologies. Many research areas and projects can be found at www.aac-rerc.com/pages/projects/projects.htm.

BioMed Central, www.biomedcentral.com
BioMed Central is an independent publishing house committed to providing immediate open access to peer-reviewed biomedical research. There is an article

titled "Intensive Language Training Enhances Brain Plasticity in Chronic Aphasia" at http://bmc.ub.uni-potsdam.de/1741-7007-2-20/.

Brain Age, www.brainage.com
The design of the Brain Age exercise program is based on the premise that cognitive exercise can improve blood flow to the brain. This Web site describes recent neurological research regarding brain training.

BrainTrain, www.braintrain.com/main/cognitive_training_research.htm
This company offers a set of brain exercises to improve attention, self-control, listening skills, reasoning ability, and memory. On their Web site, they provide an extensive number of research studies that support the basis of their programs.

Center for Applied Special Technology (CAST), www.cast.org
In research projects funded by private foundations, states, and federal agencies, CAST explores Universal Design for Learning-based solutions to education's most difficult challenges. CAST produced a document that reviews many of the technology tools for assisting students with reading and writing in grades K-8. It includes an extensive discussion and review of text modifications and innovative technology tools that alter or add to the features of printed text. Examples include text-to-speech, hypertext, and multimedia applications; spell checkers; word processors; word prediction software; word recognition software; and computer and software programs. It can be found at the following Web site: www.cast.org/publications/ncac/ncac_textrans.html#evidence.

International Dyslexia Association, www.interdys.org
The International Dyslexia Association (IDA) is a nonprofit organization dedicated to helping individuals with dyslexia and the families and communities that support them. This site reviews reading research reports.

Journal of Special Education Technology, http://jset.unlv.edu
This is a great resource to review research findings.

Kurzweil Education Systems, www.kurzweiledu.com/research.aspx
Kurzweil offers a number of software products that are very helpful for people with learning disabilities and low vision to improve learning and reading. Their Web site describes four efficacy studies that follow the development and impact Kurzweil 3000 has made in the lives of students.

The National Assistive Technology Research Institute (NATRI), natri.uky.edu
The National Assistive Technology Research Institute is currently researching the use of assistive technology. This Web site offers an opportunity to participate as well as learn what they are finding.

National Center for Technology Innovation (NATI), ww.nationaltechcenter.org
NATI is funded by the U.S. Office of Special Education Programs (OSEP). It advances learning opportunities for individuals with disabilities by fostering technology innovation and seeks to broaden and enrich the field by providing resources and promoting partnerships for the development of tools and applications by developers, manufacturers, producers, publishers, and researchers.

National Center for the Dissemination of Disability Research, www.ncddr.org
The Southwest Educational Development Laboratory (SEDL) operates the National Center for the Dissemination of Disability Research (NCDDR) through funding from the National Institute on Disability and Rehabilitation Research (NIDRR). The NCDDR scope of work responds directly to NIDRR's concern for increasing the effective use of NIDRR-sponsored research results in shaping new technologies, improving service delivery, and expanding decision-making options for people with disabilities and their families.

National Institute on Disability and Rehabilitation Research (NIDRR), www.ed.gov/about/offices/list/osers/nidrr/index.html
The National Institute on Disability and Rehabilitation Research (NIDRR) provides leadership and support for a comprehensive program of research related to the rehabilitation of individuals with disabilities.

National Rehabilitation Information Center (NARIC), www.naric.com/research
NARIC offers several products and services to researchers, practitioners, and the public. More than seventy thousand resources are gathered and made available through an easy-to-use interface. REHABDATA is a NARIC database that contains approximately sixty-nine thousand abstracts of books, reports, articles, and audiovisual materials relating to disability and rehabilitation research. Each abstract includes bibliographic information, a 250-word abstract, and, when appropriate, information regarding the project that produced the document. The index spans research from 1956 to the present.

The Traumatic Brain Injury National Data Center (TBINDC), www.tbindc.org/registry/about_registry.php
This site reviews research projects and conference presentations from the Second Federal TBI Interagency Conference in Bethesda, Maryland, in March 2006. Two interesting studies on this Web site are "MRI Changes with Cognitive Rehabilitation in Traumatic Brain Injury (TBI)" and "Principles of Neuroplasticity after Brain Injury: A Glimmer of Hope from Animal Models of Recovery."

The National Assistive Technology Research Institute, http://natri.uky.edu
The National Assistive Technology Research Institute is currently researching the use of assistive technology. This Web site offers an opportunity to participate as well as learn what they are finding.

Chapter 9:
Treatment and Technology To Improve Verbal Expression

A multimedia approach using sound, text, and pictures helps with verbal communication, learning, and recovery. Clients can benefit from the increased practice time with computers once they can repeat sounds and words from the voice output of computer programs. If they're not able to use the computer or a particular program independently, a caregiver or computer buddy should be trained to provide assistance as needed for productive home practice sessions. It's essential to analyze what helps to improve verbal expression as well as to evaluate the nature of the major obstacles. In this chapter, software is highlighted which can enhance treatment to improve verbal expression. Most selections are appropriate for all ages unless specific ages are mentioned.

In addition to exploring the use of technology to assist with improved talking, it is also important to use conventional strategies for helping people who struggle to make themselves understood. Simple steps such as providing additional response time and accepting shortened or alternative types of responses can help. People appreciate being given enough time to formulate and to speak their comments.

Verbal expression deficits can be the result of motor, structural, and pragmatic impairments from injuries or disorders:

- Stroke

- Head injury

- Aphasia

- Apraxia

- Dysarthria

- Dementia

- Progressive neurologic disease

- Developmental delay

- Language and learning disability

- Cleft palate

- Autism

- Foreign accent

- Learning English as a second language

- Hearing loss

- Voice disorder

- Intubation

Many specialized software programs, as well as mainstream products, can be used to help clients with different needs. A great deal of software is available to help improve articulation, word retrieval, sentence formulation, and dialogue. Some products are very structured, provide feedback, and are intuitive in terms of the increasing level of difficulty. There are also software programs designed to augment communication. These programs and dedicated communication devices are discussed in Chapter 9, "Additional Tools and Resources To Improve Verbal Expression."

E-books, software to make calendars, online greeting cards, calendars, newspaper programs and multimedia creative art as well as talking book programs that use graphics, text, video, voice recording, and sound can also be effective technology tools to work with during speech therapy to improve verbal expression. Chapter 15 presents multi-media programs and programs to generate printed treatment materials that can be used to improve verbal expression. Chapter 16 reviews many games and free online interactive activities that can be used to work on improving expressive speech and language.

Software Program Characteristics for Speech Goals

People who have dysarthria (slurred speech), a heavy foreign accent, verbal apraxia (speech-motor programming problems), developmental articulation errors, or impaired speech due to hearing impairments can benefit from software products for improving speech patterns. These products focus on the production of particular sounds in varying lengths of utterances. Some software describes physically how to form the sounds. Some also feature pictures of up-close mouth movements or a graphic representation of sound.

Auditory Presentation

Most of the software aimed at improving speech sound production provides recordings of the sounds for users to listen to and repeat. Some of these programs are organized by the sound to be practiced, while others present common words or words in functional contexts.

Modifying Practice With Software

Speech tasks can be varied by having the client produce multiple repetitions of a sound, syllable, or word; read words, phrases or sentences aloud, or name pictures that contain the target sounds.

Voice Recordings

There are products that record and play back the user's speech. For some clients who are unable to perceive the accuracy of their responses, this is very helpful. For others, this feature serves as a distraction.

Voice Recognition

Some of the more advanced software programs employ voice recognition. The user speaks into a microphone. Some programs convert the speech to text while others provide feedback on the accuracy of the user's speech.

Visual Biofeedback

There is software that provides computer-based visual biofeedback for pitch, volume, intonation pattern, easy onset of phonation, and articulatory precision. The programs may display waveforms and other graphic representations of verbal utterances.

Text Readers and Talking Word Processors

In addition to using software that features drill-and-practice techniques to improve speech sound production, the use of text readers and talking word processors can be very helpful. Word and sentence lists can be written into documents that the computer reads aloud. Users can practice reading aloud and then listen to the computer for help as needed or to check their responses. This type of software is described in detail in Chapter 11, "Treatment and Technology To Improve Reading Comprehension."

Software Program Characteristics for Language Goals

People who have aphasia, word-retrieval problems, delayed language, or who are learning English as a second language need to work on thinking of words as well as saying them. They also need to practice using words in phrases or sentences to convey meaning.

Software products that are helpful for improving expressive language focus on tasks involving confrontation naming, repetition and sentence formulation. The stimuli are often arranged by topic or situation rather than sounds. Some use text only, some use pictures alone or pictures with text, and others have authoring capability, so that the user or clinician can use personalized information to practice.

Many moderately impaired clients are able to communicate their basic needs and wants, repeat long sentences, and name basic pictures. These clients may have difficulty communicating more complex desires, retrieving words, and formulating sentences or abstract thoughts. When working with these more advanced clients, it is helpful to focus on challenging tasks such as:

- Recalling less common words or those with a cognitive component such as opposites or analogies

- Formulating novel sentence to describe complex pictures, steps in a task, or solutions to problems

- Engaging in dialogue for conversation-level practice

Assistive Strategies and Technology for Basic Verbal Expressive Needs

People who have had a severe stroke or head injury, vocal surgery, intubation, significant developmental delays, autism, or congenital problems, or who have limited English proficiency may have severe verbal expression problems. If a person is unable to convey basic thoughts and needs, an appropriate first goal is to find a way for them to express basic needs and wants.

It is necessary to analyze the following factors:

- The initiative the client shows in attempting to communicate

- The frequency, range of intent, and effectiveness of messages being communicated nonverbally

- The effect of cognitive, motor, and/or sensory impairments on the client's ability to learn and use nonverbal communication methods

- The resourcefulness of the communication partner to stimulate communication and understand what's expressed by the client

Voice Output Devices

Voice output devices are also referred to in the literature as AAC, augcom, and VOCA-voice-output communication aides. Once clients are able to indicate basic needs with the help of their communication partner, the next step is to consider devices that may enable clients to be more independent in their ability to select a picture or word on a communication board or in a book, or said aloud by a device.

It is helpful to look at the person's ability to generate novel verbal utterances rather than just selecting one item with the use of either pictures or words. There are low-level papers and books that picture basic need items, while others offer more words, but are also more visually complex. Voice output devices may provide a single layer of items for direct selection, while others provide multiple layers through dynamic display. Picture communication dictionaries, several of the talking Franklin products, calendars, and even address books on cell phones can also assist with communication. These will be discussed later in this chapter.

Clients who have more of a motor-based speech problem or impaired communication due to muscular weakness generally respond favorably to the functional use of communication books and talking communication devices. Clients who have severe language-based problems such as aphasia or severe cognitive deficits that interfere with talking, unfortunately do not respond as well to using dedicated communication devices functionally. People with severe aphasia and learning issues have difficulty sequencing concepts to express thoughts and needs. Often in such cases, it's the resourcefulness and ability of the communication partner to facilitate communication that determines the effectiveness of the assistive device or communication book.

Children who have not yet developed language may benefit from these items in the process of learning language. Extensive training for both adults and children is required.

Alternate Access

People who do not have a reliable method of direct selection may benefit from using switches for alternate access. As long as a person has reliable movement of any part of his or her body—such as a foot, palm of their hand, an elbow, or even a visual gaze—a system can be set up to assist with communication.

Hands-On Therapy

When a person is unable to produce sounds and words volitionally, it's necessary to work on verbal expression skills with a hands-on approach in addition to providing a way for people to point to pictures and words to express themselves. Physical prompting for speech sounds and 1:1 feedback from a person is critical in order to stimulate speech and language. This is especially true with apraxia, and is also true when the client is unable to distinguish between correct and incorrect speech sounds.

Client Customization

Technology must be individualized and used in ways to meet the needs of a client, but alone will not cure a long-term problem. These state-of-the-art devices and approaches should be used in conjunction with other traditional methods of treatment and the input of a trained professional. Clients should not be expected on their own to be able to select the appropriate software and figure out how to use it. Even after clients are using technologies in independent practice programs, it will be necessary to obtain periodic professional guidance. The choice and type of technology will continue to change during the course of therapy as the goals and needs of the client change.

Computer Software To Help Improve Verbal Expression Grouped by Software Features

As mentioned previously, different software programs provide different ways of assisting with or compensating for verbal expression challenges. The Web sites are given for each described product to provide you with information that is more detailed regarding versions of the software, networking ability, preferred operating systems, and availability of online tutorials or demos. The prices written in this guide are generally for an individual professional version of each item. These prices will undoubtedly change, but they are included to give a ballpark estimate. Most programs are suitable for both children and adults unless specifically indicated in this review.

As with other chapters in this guide, this listing is not all-inclusive, but a good place to start. Several programs are listed more than once. This was done to simplify the process when searching for software that uses a particular approach.

As you read this list, keep in mind the features that are most helpful to a particular client. Listed below are some primary characteristics or features that might be of value:

- Close-up video of mouth movement
- Pictures, text, and sounds of common words
- Pictures shown in natural settings
- Practice on specific speech sounds
- Software to increase length of utterance and syntax
- Authoring capability
- Cognitive components
- Text readers

- Topic-based sentences, dialogue tasks, and programs encouraging verbal narrative

- Visual or graphic feedback of speech and voice production

- Voice recognition

Here is a list of the order software is mentioned in this section of the chapter:

Title	Web Site	Price	PC	Mac	Online
Speech Practice	www.wingoglobal.com	$30.00	x	x	
Speech Sounds on Cue	www.bungalowsoftware.com	$199.00	x		
CHAT	www.aphasia-therapy.com	$169.50	x	x	
"It's a..." Bundle	www.learningfundamentals.com	$99.00	x	x	
Rosetta Stone English Level 1	www.rosettastone.com	$99.00	x	x	x
Talking Series	www.laureatelearning.com	$150.00	x	x	
The Great Action Adventure	www.silverliningmm.com	$69.95	x	x	
Multi-Sensory Words	www.parrotsoftware.com	Per month $24.95	x		x
Looking for Words	www.attainmentcompany.com	$99.00	x	x	
My School Day	www.silverliningmm.com	$89.99	x	x	
Talk Now! American English	www.multilinguialbooks.com	$45.00	x	x	

Title	Web Site	Price	PC	Mac	Online
Tell ME More English	www.auralog.com	CDs $195.00 Per month online $75.00	x		x
World Talk English	www.multilingualbooks.com www.best buy.com bundled in Instant Immersion English Vol. 2	$49.00 $9.95	x	x	
Sights 'n Sounds	www.bungalowsoftware.com	$199.50	x		
Articulation I, II and III	www.learningfundamentals.com	$199.50	x	x	
American Speech Sounds	www.speechcom.com	$299.00	x		
HearSay for All	www.comdistec.com	$75.00	x		
Pronunciation Power I	www. Englishlearning.com	Per year $145.00 Per month online $49.70	x		x
CHAT	www.aphasia-therapy.com	$169.50	x	x	
Language Links	www.laureatelearning.com	$195.00	x	x	
Word Order	www.parrotsoftware.com	Per month $29.95	x		
World Talk English	www.multilingualbooks.com www.bestbuy.com	$49.00 $9.95	x	x	
Clicker 5	www.cricksoft.com	$199.99	x	x	
Sights 'n Sounds	www.bungalowsoftware.com	$199.50	x		
WordPower	www.mayer-johnson	$350.00	x	x	

Title	Web Site	Price	PC	Mac	Online
Parrot Software	www.parrotsoftware.com	Per month $24.95			x
Aphasia Tutor 1 Out:Loud	www.bungalowsoftware.com	$199.00	x		
Aphasia Tutor 2 Out:Loud	www.bungalowsoftware.com	$199.00	x		
CHAT	www.aphasia-therapy.com	$169.59	x	x	
Rosetta Stone English 1	www.rosettastone.com	$195.00	x	x	x

Video of Mouth Movement

Title	Web Site	Price	PC	Mac
Speech Therapy and Speech Practice	www.wingoglobal.com	$30.00	x	x
Speech Sounds on Cue	www.bungalowsoftware.com	$199.50	x	

Many clients with aphasia, apraxia, and dysarthria greatly benefit from an up-close view of mouth movement. Some of the software programs with this feature are:

Speech Therapy CD and Speech Practice CD
by Wingo Global, www.wingoglobal.com

- These CDs were developed by Winston Lindsley, a former client of IST, and shows the mouth movement of Karen Scoggins, a former employee of IST. They require little computer interaction.

- Speech Therapy is a series of video recordings of up-close views of a model's mouth movement during expression of utterances such as counting and reciting days of the week and months of the year. The CD also has phrase completions, opposites, and carrier phrase sentences. The words are printed as the words are said aloud.

- Speech Practice focuses on the production of individual sounds and syllables.

- Specific lessons can be selected and the pause button can be pressed as needed.

- Both programs are included on one DVD for $30.00.

Speech Sounds on Cue
by Bungalow Software, www.bungalowsoftware.com

- The user first selects the target sound for practice. The software then provides drill and practice on sounds beginning with that sound in a sentence completion task with text, sound, picture, and mouth movement.

- The speaker has an Australian accent.

- Windows

- $199.50

Repetition and Naming Drill-and-Practice Tasks

Title	Web Site	Price	PC	Mac	Online
CHAT	www.aphasia-therapy.com	$169.50	x	x	
"It's a…" Bundle:	www.learningfundamentals.com	$99.00	x	x	
Rosetta Stone English	www.rosettastone.com	195.00	x	x	
Talking Series	www.laureatelearning.com	$150.00	x	x	
The Great Action Adventure	www.silverliningmm.com	$69.95	x	x	
Multi-Sensory Words	www.parrotsoftware.com	CD $99.95 Per month online $24.05	x		x

CHAT (Computerized Home Aphasia Therapy)
by Aphasia Therapy Products, www.aphasia-therapy.com

- Sounds, words, phrases, and sentences are presented in text form and are read aloud by both a man's and a woman's voice.

- CHAT provides extensive opportunities for repetition as well as word retrieval in a wide variety of carefully controlled tasks.

- It's very intuitive and straightforward for clients to use at home for independent practice.

- There is a unique section with Melodic Intonation Training, which displays notes on a treble clef along with the audio and text if desired.

- Most lessons at the initial levels progress at a preprogrammed rate with no clicking. The more difficult levels, which work on word retrieval, allow the client to control the rate at which the items are presented.

- Voice cannot be recorded and there are no options within a lesson. Feedback regarding accuracy of performance is not given.

- Windows and Mac

- $169.50

"It's a…" Bundle: Therapy for Expressive Naming Disorders
by Learning Fundamentals, www.learningfundamentals.com

- This bundle has three programs.

- The first program has 100 pictures of food, 100 pictures of everyday objects, 100 mixed pictures, 120 pictures of animals in their habitats, and 25 pictures of Spanish foods.

- The program "And a One, Two, Three!" focuses on syllable segmentation practice.

- There are a variety of cueing strategies to provide both visual confrontation and responsive naming tasks. Voice can be recorded.

- Windows and Mac

- $99.00

Rosetta Stone English
by Rosetta Stone, www.rosettastone.com

- This program spans the range of very basic tasks to quite complex.

- The verbal expression modality can be selected by clicking the microphone. There are also exercises to work on listening, reading, and writing.

- The initial verbal expression lessons include confrontation-naming tasks. Lessons that are more difficult work on sentence formulation.

- The user's voice is recorded and played back with the target utterance. A graded meter assesses the perceived accuracy of the response, and a voiceprint is provided.

- This software is available in twenty-nine languages.

- Windows and Mac

- The Level 1 English CD is $195.00. There is also an online version. The price varies with the length of time purchased.

Talking Series
by Laureate Learning Systems, www.laureatelearning.com

- This program is helpful when trying to figure out whether a client is an appropriate candidate for a dedicated communication device.

- There are three programs in this series—Talking Nouns 1, Talking Nouns 2, and Talking Verbs—with about fifty stimuli each.

- The therapist first selects the words to be provided and the nature of the task.

- With the "interactive communication" selection, the computer can either be set to say each word as it is selected or to speak only after a phrase or sentence has been completed. In both cases, the computer adds articles and verb inflections so that only grammatically correct phrases are heard.

- In the picture-matching task, a picture appears on the monitor and the user is asked to find its match.

- In the picture-identification task, the computer names a picture and the user finds it.

- Animation is provided on the Talking Verbs CD.

- Windows and Mac

- $150.00 – Families receive a 50 percent discount.

The Great Action Adventure
by Silver Lining Multimedia, www.silverliningmm.com

- Skills taught include receptive noun and verb matching, sign language, word matching, and verb tenses.

- This software is most appropriate for children.

- It includes full-motion video of verbs and sign language.

- The lessons are customizable with both play and learning areas. The clinician selects which words are taught, how they are presented, and how the student is reinforced and prompted.

- Windows and Mac

- $69.95

Multi-Sensory Words
by Parrot Software, www.parrotsoftware.com

- A picture is displayed, and the user is asked to say or write its name.
- The response can be recorded for playback.
- If the "Hear Word" icon is pressed, a voice says the word.
- The client can choose to see the first letter of the word or to see or hear the entire word as needed.
- Windows
- This program is part of the online Parrot subscription for $24.95 a month or it can be purchased individually for $99.95.

Words in Natural Settings

It is often helpful for clients with language deficits to see pictures of items in context or grouped by category. In addition to using the following programs to create drill-and-practice opportunities for language activities, a creative therapist might be able to encourage the client to use the following programs to facilitate communication. Several of these programs are meant to be used as language courses to teach English. They offer a vast array of lessons based on different functional topics.

Title	Web Site	Price	PC	Mac	Online
Language Activities of Daily Living	www.laureatelearning.com	$150.00	x	x	
Looking for Words	www.attainmentcompany.com	$99.00	x	x	
My School Day	www.silverliningmm.com	$89.99	x	x	
Talk Now! American English	www.multilinguialbooks.com	$45.00	x	x	
Tell ME More English	www.auralog.com	CDs $195.00 Per month online $75.00	x		x
World Talk English	www.multilingualbooks.com	$49.00	x	x	

Title	Web Site	Price	PC	Mac	Online
	www.best buy.com bundled in Instant Immersion English Vol. 2	$9.95			

Language Activities of Daily Living: My House, My Town, and My School
by Laureate Learning Systems, www.laureatelearning.com

- These programs offer house, town, and school environments in which children and adults learn about objects and activities encountered in daily living routines.

- Each program includes six scenes to teach over one hundred common vocabulary items.

- In the My House CD, the software presents vocabulary items found in the living room, dining room, kitchen, bedroom, bathroom, and utility room.

- The My Town CD works with vocabulary items found in the doctor's office, dentist's office, restaurant, park, city neighborhood, and suburban neighborhood.

- The My School CD presents vocabulary in the classroom, playground, cafeteria, library, music/art room, and hallway.

- There are four activities for each scene. The user can click on an object, and the computer says its name or function. There are also activities in which the user asks the user to find the location of a named or described object.

- Client customization is encouraged. Clients can click on pictures and hear the names spoken aloud, they can work on repetition, or they can practice naming items first without hearing or reading the names.

- To develop verbal expression that is more complex, the therapist can have the client use the word in a sentence, practice multiple repetitions, or formulate clues to have the clinician find the described item.

- Windows and Mac

- $150.00

Looking for Words
by Attainment Company, www.attainmentcompany.com

- This program presents three different settings to explore: the home, the town, and the school.

- The cursor turns into a magnifying glass in the explore mode. It is possible to enter different rooms in a house and go to different streets in a town. Once in a location, an item is selected and then highlighted. The text is printed in large letters while the item is named aloud.

- This is great for confrontation naming as well as repetition. When it's too easy to repeat the word, the task can be made more difficult by having the client repeat it multiple times or use the word in a sentence.

- This software also has a task in which the user finds items on a list, which involves memory, sequencing, and reasoning. Verbal expression skills can be practiced during this task by having clients verbalize where they are going, why, and what they will do next to find items on the list.

- Windows and Mac

- $99.00

My School Day
by Silver Lining Multimedia, www.silverliningmm.com

- My School Day uses real-life video to take the child into a typical school day, including the classroom, cafeteria, and playground.

- It provides an opportunity for students to view appropriate interactions and social behaviors within the school environment.

- The user is asked to identify, produce, and explain several social situations in response to the video, which is embedded in interactive software.

- Progress can be charted.

- It's appropriate for children with the cognitive ages of six to fifteen years old.

- Windows and Mac

- $89.99

Talk Now! American English
by EuroTalk, available for purchase in the United States at
www.multilingualbooks.com.

It is also bundled into Instant Immersion English Vol. 2, which is available at
www.bestbuy.com or www.amazon.com.

- To work on verbal expression skills, the user first selects a category. Categories include basic phrases, colors, numbers, food, shopping, and time. Clients can practice repeating and naming pictured items.

- There are hundreds of items to practice in a game format and several ways to work on saying the names of pictures. Users can name items and then click to hear the word and compare it to the correct production. There is also a game in which users name a set number of items in a row and then record their utterances.

- This software is available in 102 languages.

- Windows and Mac

- $45.00

Tell Me More English
by Auralog, www.auralog.com

- This program is divided into six workshops.

- The Grammar and Vocabulary Workshop include sets of exercises linked to grammar rules, verb conjugations, and key vocabulary words (classified by either topic or level.)

- The Oral Workshop contains numerous dialogues and interactive videos focusing on both oral comprehension and expression.

- The Dynamic Mode uses real-time performance analysis to tailor the English-learning process based on results.

- The Guided Mode offers a personalized lesson structure based on objectives and time constraints.

- The Free-to-Roam Mode allows the user to select activities and workshops.

- Speech recognition technology evaluates pronunciation, and detects and corrects errors.

- 3-D animations illustrate the movements of the lips and mouth.

- Both CD and online formats are available in English (American and British), Spanish, German, French, Italian, Dutch, Chinese, Japanese, and Arabic.

- Windows and Online

- Several CD and customized subscriptions for online versions are available. The "month pass" is $75. The Tell Me More Premium CD collection is $195.

World Talk English
by EuroTalk, is available at www.multilingualbooks.com.

- It is also bundled into Instant Immersion English Vol. 2, which is available at www.bestbuy.com or www.amazon.com.

- There are ten interactive games to play featuring topics such as food, weather, directions, sentence construction, and animals.

- A "Recording Studio" can be used for practicing verbal expression, sentence construction, and word retrieval.

- In the section "Word Practice," the computer pronounces selected words and the user can imitate them. Alternately, the user can try to say them first and then click on the words as needed for support.

- In the section "Speaking Practice," the computer pronounces the names of a sequence of pictures. Users select an icon with the microphone and record their pronunciation of these items.

- This software is available in many languages.

- Windows and Mac

- $49.00

Repetition Tasks With Stimuli Grouped by Speech Sound

Software to help with articulation of specific sounds can be divided into two distinct groups: some programs are produced for people with special needs, while others are produced for foreign accent reduction. The software designed for special needs is typically very intuitive and uses large text and graphics. These programs are often easy for clients to use for independent practice. There is generally helpful phone support as needed. Products designed for accent reduction are typically more visually challenging for people with visual-perceptual issues. Users can listen to the word said aloud as often as needed. Speech can be recorded and played back for comparison to the recorded computer voice. These programs are very helpful for clients who have apraxia and dysarthria, as well as for people who are working on improving clarity and fluency of connected speech.

Title	Web site	Price	PC	Mac	Online
American Speech Sounds	www.speechcom.com	$149.95	x		

Title	Web site	Price	PC	Mac	Online
Articulation I, II and III	www.learningfundamentals.com	$199.50	x	x	
Dudsberry's Fishing Fun	www.janellepublications.com	$39.00	x	x	
HearSay for All	www.comdistec.com	$75.00	x		
Pronunciation Power I	www. Englishlearning.com	$145.00 Per month online $49.70	x		x
Sights 'n Sounds	www.bungalowsoftware.com	$199.50	x		

American Speech Sounds
by Speech Com, www.speechcom.com

- The professional version includes more than eight thousand words and expressions, as well as consonants and vowels, with video and audio.

- Recordings can be made, immediate feedback is provided, and performance scores are documented.

- Lessons offer practice with fluency, intonation, and distinguishing between correctly and incorrectly produced sounds and words.

- Authoring exercises enable the therapist to create customized professional terms, names, places, slang, dialogues, and narratives.

- There is a guide for thirty different language backgrounds. This software is intended to be used for foreign accent reduction, but it's quite helpful for a wide variety of therapy to improve verbal expression.

- Video clips, diagrams, instructions, explanations of common problems, and spelling examples are presented for every sound.

- There are two versions available: one for personal use and another for users who are health-care professionals.

- Windows

- $149.95

Articulation I, II, and III
by LocuTour Multimedia, www.learningfundamentals.com

- Users can practice saying sounds, words, phrases, and sentences.

- Digitized speech presents stimuli in normal or exaggerated speech models.

- Onscreen recording and playback are provided for immediate feedback.

- Articulation I focuses on consonant phonemes, Articulation II works on consonant clusters, and Articulation III works with vowels plus /R/ and /R/ clusters.

- Windows and Mac

- $99.00

Dudsberry's Fishing Fun
by Janelle Publications, www.janellepublications.com

- Children are engaged in the adventures of a dog, named Dudsberry, who is asleep in his doghouse, then roused by a storm. His photo album is blown away and the activities help him re-build his album.

- A fishing game is used to practice saying the phonemes: r, l, s, and r, l, and s blends.

- Speech skills can be practiced at the word, sentence, and spontaneous speech level.

- There are 150 photos with Dudsberry.

- Windows and Mac

- $39.00

HearSay for All
by Communication Disorders Technology, www.comdistec.com

- HearSay provides individualized pronunciation practice using automatic speech recognition in an interactive-game environment.

- It focuses primarily on the sounds most important for speech intelligibility, and it identifies the speech sounds with which the user most often has difficulty producing when learning to speak English as a second language.

- The feedback of speech production is displayed graphically in the HearSay Progress Chart. This chart shows speaking and listening skills on over seven hundred word pairs containing contrasting sounds,

- Users select from the word pairs displayed in the chart and hear them spoken by American English speakers, or they speak them and receive evaluative feedback on their pronunciation.

- The system has a built-in training sequence that adapts automatically to the current skill level.

- Separate versions of HearSay are designed specifically for Japanese speakers, Mandarin Chinese speakers, and Spanish speakers of English.

- Windows

- $75.00

Pronunciation Power 1
by English Learning, www.englishlearning.com

- The user first selects a sound. Both front and side views are shown for all of the fifty-two sounds at normal speed and in slow motion

- Drill-and-practice exercises are given for more than seven thousand words at the word and sentence levels.

- After a sound is presented, it's followed by speech analysis activities, lessons, and four different kinds of exercises, sample words, comparative words, listening discrimination, and sentences.

- Illustrations and photographs are used to illustrate the production of sounds.

- Several other products are also available, such as Pronunciation Power 2 and Pronunciation Power Idioms.

- Pronunciation Power includes the 8-in-1 English Dictionary at no additional charge.

- The dictionary offers translations in twelve languages and over two thousand pictures and graphics. Users can listen to and record over seven thousand words, including plurals of nouns and conjugations of verbs. There are ten different ways to search for words: by themes such as animals, colors, and clothing; by the location of the sound in a word; or by whether it is a verb or a noun.

- Windows

- Three purchase scenarios are offered: a CD, download, or online subscription. The CD is $154.95 and a ninety-day Web-based subscription is $49.70.

Sights 'n Sounds
by Bungalow Software, www.bungalowsoftware.com

- This program has six lessons and over four hundred words.

- Sections include single-syllable words, short words organized by beginning sound, short words organized by ending sound, pictures and words for nouns, pictures and words for verbs, and words for abstract concepts.

- There is an authoring component to this program. This is a very helpful feature so that users can practice saying personal information such as the names of family and friends, important phrases, home phone numbers, and addresses.

- Windows
- $199.50

Software To Increase Length of Utterance and Improve Syntax

The following programs do not necessarily record voice or provide a verbal model for sentence formation. However, they are very helpful in working on lengthening a verbal response.

Title	Web Site	Price	PC	Mac
CHAT	www.aphasia-therapy.com	$169.50	x	x
Language Links	www.laureatelearning.com	$195.00	x	x
Word Order	www.parrotsoftware.com	Per month $29.95	x	
World Talk English	www.multilingualbooks.com www.bestbuy.com	$49.00 $9.95	x	x

CHAT (Computerized Home Aphasia Therapy)
by Aphasia Therapy Products, www.aphasia-therapy.com

- Sounds, words, phrases, and sentences are presented in text form and read aloud by both a man's and a woman's voice.
- There are quite a few lessons that focus on gradually increasing the length of utterance.
- Windows and Mac
- $169.50

LanguageLinks
by Laureate Learning Systems, www.laureateLearning.com

- LanguageLinks is a new, comprehensive, approach to syntax assessment and intervention.

- It takes users from the early two-word development stage through the mastery of a broad range of syntactic forms.

- Six levels train over 75 essential grammatical forms in developmental order.

- The software begins with an assessment to determine where to start training. Then the program tracks detailed information about performance and automatically guides the users through the curriculum.

- Windows and Mac

- $195.00

Word Order
by Parrot Software, www.parrotsoftware.com

- This program displays scrambled sentences.

- The user examines the words and constructs a sentence using them.

- Words are selected by clicking on them in order.

- Windows

- This program is included in the Online Parrot Subscription for $29.95 a month, $99.95 if purchased alone.

World Talk English
by EuroTalk, www.multilingualbooks.com

- World Talk is aimed at intermediate level learners.

- There are 10 interactive games to play featuring topics such as food, weather, directions, sentence construction, and animals.

- The sentence construction game presents a series of words in a sentence after a brief dialogue is heard.

- The user clicks on the words in order to form the sentence.

- This program is available in a wide variety of languages.

- Windows or Mac

- This program is bundled in the Instant Immersion English V.2 that can be found at bestbuy.com for $9.95.

Software With an Authoring Feature

Programs that offer the ability to customize the stimuli items are helpful for learning to say personalized information and for creating practice materials that are relevant for each client. Some of these programs are in a drill-and-practice format with feedback, while others provide a tool for clinicians to work with clients toward targeted goals, but don't lend themselves as well for independent client practice without feedback from another person.

Title	Web Site	Price	PC	Mac
Clicker 5	www.cricksoft.com	$199.99	x	x
Sights 'n Sounds	www.bungalowsoftware.com	$199.50	x	
WordPower	www.mayer-johnson	$350.00	x	x

Clicker 5
by Crick Software, www.cricksoft.com

- This software contains a set of grids on the bottom half of the screen. Words, phrases, or pictures can be placed in the cells of the grid.
- The program includes thousands of pictures and the grids are easy to produce.
- The lessons are either set up by the clinician or downloaded from www.learninggrids.com. The majority of the sets are designed for students from pre-school onwards. However, there is a category for adult learners that contains some sets that can be adapted and used by adults.
- Digital photos as well as video clips of items in a house or family members can be used.
- The user can right click on the pictures or words in the grid to have the computer say aloud what was recorded for that cell.
- When the cells in the grid with words or pictures are selected with a left mouse click, the contents of the cell are moved to a talking word processor on the top half of the screen.
- Several cells can be selected to form sentences. When final punctuation is used, the computer reads the sentence aloud.
- Windows and Mac
- $199.00

Sights 'n Sounds
by Bungalow Software, www.bungalowsoftware.com

- This program has six lessons and over four hundred words.

- Sections include single-syllable words, short words organized by beginning sound, short words organized by ending sound, pictures and words for nouns, pictures and words for verbs, and words for abstract concepts.

- The last lesson provides an authoring component to this program. It can be programmed so users can practice saying personal information such as the names of family and friends, important phrases, home phone numbers, and addresses.

- Digital pictures or any graphic that is in a computer file can be used to support the meaning of the text or to turn the task into a word or phrase retrieval task, as opposed to a reading aloud exercise.

- Windows

- $199.50

WordPower
by Nancy Inman, distributed by Mayer-Johnson at www.mayer-johnson.com

- WordPower combines the features of core vocabulary, spelling, and word prediction.

- The system capitalizes on the fact that a core of just one hundred words accounts for approximately 50 percent of most words spoken.

- Four components are included: WordPower (for text users), Picture WordPower (for users who need picture cues), Scanning Word Power, and Scanning Picture WordPower.

- Picture WordPower consists of single-hit words, category-based words, and spelling with word prediction. The core words are categorized, color coded, and alphabetized for easy access.

- Clients can formulate phrases and sentences by selecting pictures and then saying them aloud.

- This program needs a dedicated communication device platform on which to work. The least expensive option is also to purchase Speaking Dynamically Pro (a picture-based, text-based, augmentative, and alternative communication software sold for $359, also at www.mayer-johnson.com).

- Windows and Mac

- $350.00

Cognitive Component for Production of Novel Speech Utterances

Many higher-level clients are quite capable of performing straightforward language tasks, such as repeating sentences and naming pictures; however, when reasoning and memory components are added to the task, performance deteriorates. Deficits are often exacerbated when clients are asked to describe solutions to problems, complete analogy tasks, or summarize written material. As tasks become more abstract, the response becomes more difficult.

Parrot Software
by Parrot Software, www.parrotsoftware.com

- Parrot Software offers many cognitively based programs as part of the online subscription that can be used to improve verbal expression.

- Most responses to the drill-and-practice exercises require typing the response or selecting an item in a multiple-choice format.

- Users can verbalize responses while completing lessons that may have a multiple choice format or require a written response.

- Programs requiring higher-level language skills include Inferential Naming, Deductive Reasoning, Situational Reasoning, Things in Common, Reasons Why, Problem Solving, Cause and Effect, and Sequence of Events.

- For users with significant cognitive or visual-perceptual deficits, have a "computer buddy" access the program and get the user started on the appropriate tasks. The initial menu can be overwhelming.

- One drawback is that three clicks are often needed for responses. One click is needed for the response, another to acknowledge the computer feedback, and another to move to the next item.

- There are a large number of programs from which to choose. They are not presented in any particular order of difficulty, but they are grouped into categories.

- Phone support is excellent.

- Windows

- An online subscription is $24.95 a month. Programs can also be purchased separately.

Text-Based and Picture-Based Software Not Grouped by Sound or Topic

Title	Web site	Price	PC	Mac	Online
Aphasia Tutor 1+ Out Loud	www.bungalowsoftware.com	$199.00	x		
Aphasia Tutor 2+ Out Loud	www.bungalowsoftware.com	$199.00	x		
CHAT	www.aphasia-therapy.com	$169.59	x	x	
Rosetta Stone English 1	www.rosettastone.com	$195.00	x	x	x

Aphasia Tutor Series: (AT) 1+ Out Loud and Aphasia Tutor (AT) 2+ Out Loud
by Bungalow Software, www.bungalowsoftware.com

- AT1 and AT2 are intended for practice with reading and writing of words, phrases, and sentences.

- These programs can be used to practice word retrieval, sentence-level reading aloud, spelling, and naming.

- Lessons include phrase and sentence completions (fill-in and matching) and sentence-picture matching. Cues and answers are spoken aloud for extra help.

- Text and graphics are easy to see, and the program is easy to use for people with significant deficits. Minimal clicking is required, and alternate input devices can be used.

- Windows

- $199.00 for each professional version.

Beyond Speech Therapy
by Beyond Speech Therapy, Inc., www.beyondspeechtherapy.com

- This Web-based program enables therapists to provide a structured, intensive, personalized online speech therapy program for home practice.

- It is updated regularly, and the questions are randomized.

- The program can be delivered to hospitals, skilled nursing facilities, universities, or patients' homes.

- Programs are provided for the treatment of aphasia, apraxia, dysarthria, dysphagia, and higher-level language skills

- The site license and setup fee is $500.00

- Speech-language pathologists customize the program for each client. The fee for the client to be able to access the program at home is $34.99 a month.

CHAT (Computerized Home Aphasia Therapy)
by Aphasia Therapy Products, www.aphasia-therapy.com

- Sounds, words, phrases, and sentences are presented in text form and read aloud by both a man's and a woman's voice.

- CHAT provides extensive opportunities for repetition as well as word retrieval in a wide variety of carefully controlled tasks.

- There is a unique section with Melodic Intonation Training, which displays notes on a treble clef along with the audio and text if desired.

- Windows and Mac

- $169.50

Rosetta Stone English
by Rosetta Stone, www.rosettastone.com

- This software was produced primarily to teach English as a second language.

- The verbal expression modality can be selected by clicking the microphone.

- The initial verbal expression lessons include confrontation-naming tasks. Lessons that are more difficult work on sentence formulation.

- The user's voice is recorded and played back with the target utterance.

- A graded meter assesses the perceived accuracy of the response, and a voiceprint is provided.

- It's available in twenty-nine languages and particular aspects of grammar can be targeted.

- Windows and Mac

- The Level 1 English CD is $195. There is also an online version, whose price varies with the length of time purchased. One month online is $49.95.

Text Readers

Text-reading software reads text aloud from the computer. The multi-sensory input can be very helpful when working to improve verbal expression. Word lists, phrases, and sentences can be read aloud. Clients can practice reading text aloud, and then have the computer read it aloud for support or to check their accuracy. Many of these programs work with e-mail, Web sites, and both Word and PDF documents. Some highlight or enlarge the words as they are read aloud.

A variety of voices is available such as NEO voices, AT&T voices, Acapela voices, and Microsoft Voices. The rate of speech can be selected and changed as needed. It is important to provide opportunities for the client to select the voice, voice rate, and highlighting features that work best for them. Many clients with communication and cognitive deficits greatly benefit from a slower rate of speech. Once the skill has been mastered, the appropriate options selected, and stimuli presented to the user, effective treatment can be provided.

More information about text readers and how they can integrate into treatment can be found in Chapter 12, "Treatment and Technology To Improve Reading Comprehension."

Here are a few examples of text readers:

- Universal Reader by Premiere Assistive Technology at www.readingmadeeasy.com

- NextUp Talker at www.nextup.com

- WordQ by Quillsoft at www.wordq.com

Topic-Based Sentences, Dialogue Tasks, and Programs Encouraging Verbal Narrative

Many clients need help establishing carryover with new articulatory patterns, fluent speech, word retrieval strategies, and the organization of content in connected discourse. A computer can be used as a context for this type of practice in many ways. The therapist or a computer buddy can provide communication models and work toward verbal communication goals while using engaging activities with the client on the computer. Games can be used as discussed in Chapter 16, Multi-media programs can be used as discussed in Chapter 15 and many of the resources mentioned in Chapter 9 can be used to encourage verbal narrative.

High-level clients can also benefit from many non-tech-related solutions in order to practice the following conversational skills:

- Aphasia Groups, www.aphasia.org

- Book clubs — Reading for Life, www.readinggroupguides.com

- Toastmaster's International, www.toastmasters.org

Additional activities to work on verbal expression skills may include the following:

- Playing games

- Producing online greeting cards

- Writing stories

- Composing e-mail messages and instant messages and participating in chat rooms

- Reviewing trip-planning Web sites

Visual/Graphic Feedback of Speech and Voice Production

Title	Web Site	Price	PC	Mac
Dr. Speech	www.drspeech.com	$295.00	x	
Soliloquy Reading Assistant	www.soliloquylearning.com	$229.00	x	x
Sona-Speech II, Model 3650	www.kayelemetrics.com	Talk to Representative	x	
Sound Beginning 1	www.turningpointtechnology.com	$69.95	x	
Sound Beginning 2	www.toolfactory.com	$69.95	x	
TalkTime with Tucker	www.laureatelearning.com	$125.00	x	x
Tiger's Tale	www.laureatelearning.com	$125	X	x
Video Voice Speech Training System	www.videovoice.com	$995.00	x	

Dr. Speech
by Tiger DRS, www.drspeech.com

- Dr. Speech software is a portable speech/voice assessment and training software system.

- The Speech Therapy product uses over thirty voice-activated video games to provide real-time reinforcement of a client's attempts to produce changes in pitch, loudness, voiced and unvoiced phonation, voicing onset, maximum phonation time, sound, and vowel tracking.

- Due to the animated feedback, this program is most appropriate for children.

- The program works on both awareness and skill-building activities.

- User logs track progress.

- Windows

- Speech Therapy Basic costs $295.00

- Speech Therapy, a more complete version with assessment and printout functions, costs $695.00

Soliloquy Reading Assistant
by Soliloquy Learning, Inc. at http://www.soliloquylearning.com

- This program provides computer interactive guided oral reading.

- Soliloquy Reading Assistant combines speech recognition and verification technology with reading research and educational science to help individuals develop fluency.

- As the user reads aloud a story from one of the anthologies into a headset microphone, Soliloquy Reading Assistant "listens" along, guiding the user through the text and providing audio and visual help for difficult words.

- The program provides a review list of all words for which the user received assistance.

- Quiz questions test comprehension

- Windows and Mac

- $229.00

Sona-Speech II, Model 3650
by KayPENTAX, www.kayelemetrics.com

- Sona-Speech II software is used as a therapy tool for a broad range of speech and voice problems.

- It provides real-time visual feedback of important speech/voice parameters and quantitative measurements to track performance.

- There are eight separate modules designed for assessment and treatment of voice, articulation, fluency, motor speech (dysarthria), and other communication disorders.

- It provides graphically interesting games.

- Windows

- Pricing is offered in conjunction with individual consultation with a sales representative.

Sound Beginnings 1
by Tool Factory at www.turningpointtechnology.com

- Using a microphone, the user follows directions and controls the actions of characters on the screen.

- The teacher options include printable student records, configuration controls for speed and frequency, and the ability to import pictures and photos within the Jigsaw activity.

- There are five voice-controlled activities:

  - Jigsaw puzzle

  - Jumping creature who responds to vocalized commands

  - Blow Up Balloon - The longer you speak the bigger the balloon gets.

  - Pitch Game - The pitch of your voice controls the player's movements.

  - Space Game - Beat the enemy by saying "Fire," "Left," or "Right."

- Windows

- $69.95

Sound Beginnings 2
by Tool Factory at www.tooltime.com

- The user uses a microphone to control characters and games with voice.

- Activities offer several levels and can be configured. They include:

  - Counting - Students count characters from one to ten.

  - Flying - Sustain a sound to keep a creature floating in the sky.

  - Painting - Paint a picture by using noise or speech.

  - Racing - Use sustained sound and volume to race a car.

  - Placing - Use placement words to place a character in a room.

- Most appropriate for children

- Windows

- $69.95

TalkTime with Tucker
by Laureate Learning Systems, www.laureatelearning.com

- This voice-activated program encourages children with speech impairments to vocalize.

- When the child talks or makes sounds into the microphone, Tucker moves and talks. This program accepts a broad range of sounds and speech to make Tucker come alive. Almost any input is followed by an appropriate response.

- There are activities to teach cause and effect, turn-taking, animal sound imitation, increasing verbalization length, changing voice volume, and natural communication exchanges.

- Windows and Mac

- $125.00

Tiger's Tale
by Laureate Learning Systems, www.laureatelearning.com

- It pediatric oriented program stimulates language production by encouraging students to "talk" for a tiger that has lost his voice. Preschool and elementary students are motivated by recording their voices to create their own movies.

- During the tiger's search, animated characters appear and ask children questions to elicit their thoughts, suggestions, and opinions.

- These "home" movies, which can be saved for future viewing, are enjoyable to watch and can help measure progress over time.

- Windows and Mac

- $125.00

Video Voice Speech Training System 3.0
by Micro Video Corporation, www.videovoice.com

- Video Voice offers a wide variety of entertaining, motivational graphic display, and game formats that have many applications for developing speech skills with both children and adults.

- This new, software-only system requires only a microphone to use.

- Windows

- The price for a single computer is $995.00.

Voice Recognition

One type of voice recognition software is used often in mainstream society to enable the computer to type what is said aloud. Here are two examples:

- Dragon Naturally Speaking by Nuance, www.nuance.com
- Speech recognition built-into Microsoft Word 2003 and Microsoft Windows XP

Clients with cognitive and verbal expression deficits often have difficulty using these products successfully. It's important for clients to understand that computer-based feedback is not always consistent with human-based perceptions. The computer is not always right. Training is difficult for people with communication deficits because they have to read lengthy passages aloud. It is also necessary to remember multiple verbal commands to use and to be able to perform a sequence of steps to correct errors made by the computer to improve its accuracy.

Voice recognition software is most helpful with clients who present with written expression deficits due to motor issues or people who have visual perceptual deficits. More information can be found in Chapter 12, "Treatment and Technology To Improve Written Expression."

Quite a few software programs incorporate voice-recognition features to provide feedback regarding the accuracy of a verbal response. Examples include:

Title	Web Site	Price	PC	Mac	Online
Mastering Personal Information	www.parrotsoftware.com	$99.95 Per month online $24.95	x		x
Say a Suitable Adjective	www.parrotsoftware.com	$99.95 Per month online $24.95	x		x
Scrambled Sentences: Say It	www.parrotsoftware.com	$99.95 Per month online $24.95	x		x
SpeakQ	www.quillsoft.com	With WordQ $350.00	x		
Tell Me More English	www.auralog.com	CDs $195.00 Per month online $75.00	x		x

Title	Web Site	Price	PC	Mac	Online
Using Prepositions	www.parrotsoftware.com	$99.95 Per month online $24.95	x		x
Using Propositional Speech	www.parrotsoftware.com	$99.95 Per month online $24.95	x		x

Mastering Personal Information
by Parrot Software, www.parrotsoftware.com

- Users are asked to provide pieces of information by typing or writing the information.
- $99.95 or online subscription for $24.95 a month

Say a Suitable Adjective
by Parrot Software, www.parrotsoftware.com

- Users describe the shape, color, and size of geometric forms.
- $99.95 or online subscription for $24.95 a month

Scrambled Sentences: Say It
by Parrot Software, www.parrotsoftware.com

- Users are presented with words in a sentence and are asked to speak the sentences in the correct order.
- $99.95 or online subscription for $24.95 a month

SpeakQ
by Quillsoft, www.quillsoft.com

- This is a relatively new voice-recognition product developed for users with mild-to-moderate communication and cognitive deficits.
- It is easier to use than other speech-recognition products developed to write what is said aloud because it does not require fluent, clear speech or the ability to remember multiple commands.
- After the software has been trained to recognize the client's speech, it can be used in therapy to practice saying words and utterances and trying to get the computer to type what is said.

- SpeakQ plugs into WordQ and adds simple speech recognition. It features a simple training interface by which the computer prompts the user by voice in what to say.

- The users can then dictate directly into any document or dictate into WordQ's prediction list. Speech is combined with the word prediction.

- To keep it simple, there are no verbal commands; the user only dictates text.

- Windows

- The WordQ and SpeakQ bundle costs $350.

Tell Me More English
by Auralog, www.auralog.com

- This program, which was described earlier in this chapter, has a component in which the computer uses a visual meter to grade the accuracy of the verbal response.

Using Prepositions
by Parrot Software, www.parrotsoftware.com

- Users move pictures from the left side of the screen to the right side by using a command that mentions both the name of the pictures and the new locations.

- Windows

- $99.95 or online subscription for $24.95 a month

Using Propositional Speech
by Parrot Software, www.parrotsoftware.com

- Users are presented with a grid of pictures on the left side of the screen and must give a verbal command to place the pictures in a predetermined place on the right side.

- Windows

- $99.95 or online subscription for $24.95 a month

Chapter 10:
Additional Tools and Resources To Help Improve Verbal Expression

There are many tools and resources that can be used to help improve verbal expression in addition to the wide variety of software presented in Chapter 8, "Treatment and Technology To Improve Verbal Expression." Augmentative and Alternative Communication (AAC) is the field that focuses on helping individuals whose speech does not meet their communication needs. Consistency with treatment and training on the use of these tools is the key to the successful integration of them into the client's daily life.

Many types of devices and assistive communication tools and strategies can be used to facilitate expressive communication:

- Simple communication items without voice output
- Dedicated communication devices
- Direct-select, one-level, voice output communication devices
- Multiple-level, voice output devices
- Dynamic display, voice output devices
- Communication software that can be used on the client's computer
- Devices and software that use a client's own speech to clarify the message
- Telephones, videophones, and assistive options
- Music
- Training communication partners

Simple Communication Items Without Voice Output

Clinicians can support spoken responses by providing symbols, pictures, or words that the client selects. Books, picture communication charts, calendars, maps, and other items help augment expressive communication. The term "symbols" in AAC refers to both unaided symbols and aided symbols. Unaided symbols include gestures, facial expressions, sign language, and body posture. Aided symbols include objects, photographs, line drawings, picture communication symbols, and the alphabet. These simple communication items without voice output are very helpful in therapy, both for individual and group sessions. Families should be encouraged to personalize the content as much as possible. In addition to using these types of materials to augment communication, they can be used to have clients read aloud, name, and sequence pictures to form messages. Auditory comprehension and reasoning tasks can also be created with these products.

Title	Web Site	Price
Critical Communicator	www.interactivetherapy.com	$23.00
Daily Communicator	www.interactivetherapy.com	Approx. $25.00
Oxford Picture Dictionary: Monolingual English Edition	available at www.amazon.com and other bookstores	$14.95
Oxford Picture Dictionary for the Content Areas—Monolingual English	available at www.amazon.com and other bookstores	$14.25
SparkChart on ESL Vocabulary	www.sparkcharts.com	$4.95
Topic Boards	www. Communication-innovations.com	$5.00
Vidatak E-Z Board	www.vidatak.com	$16.50

Critical Communicator (Revised)
by Interactive Therapeutics, www.interactivetherapy.com

- The Critical Communicator is a word-and-picture communication board. Basic care concepts are provided in an easy-to-use menu format.

- It is appropriate for use with patients in critical care settings, such as ICU, trauma units, emergency departments, specialized ventilator units, post-surgery areas, long-term care, home health, and hospices.

- There are twenty-five communication boards per package, and they are available in English or Spanish for $23.00.

Critical Communicator for Kids
by Interactive Therapeutics, www.interactivetherapy.com

- This child-friendly word-and-picture communication board includes foods, activities, and toys, as well as a pain scale and other needs.

- The board can be used to assist family and staff to interact with children who need help communicating on a temporary basis.

- It's helpful in post-surgery areas, emergency rooms, intensive care, and trauma and specialized units.

- A pack of twenty-five copies on heavy 8½ × 11-inch card stock is available in English or Spanish for $23.00.

Daily Communicator
by Interactive Therapeutics, www.interactivetherapy.com

- Interactive Therapeutics offers a variety of small-ring or large-ring binders that have categorized lists with tabs, printed on sturdy card stock.

- Categories include topics such as About Me, Basic Needs, Meal Needs, Action Words, and Feelings. Both pictures and words can be used.

- The price is approximately $25.00. Supplemental packs can be purchased, and a Spanish version is available.

The Oxford Picture Dictionary: Monolingual English Edition
by Jayme Adelson-Goldstein and Norma Shapiro, available at www.amazon.com and other bookstores

- This dictionary includes 3,600 words subdivided into 140 different topics (fruits, anatomy, geography, and so on), with detailed, full-color illustrations.
- $14.95

The Oxford Picture Dictionary for the Content Areas—Monolingual English
by Jayme Adelson-Goldstein and Norma Shapiro, available at www.amazon.com and other bookstores

- The dictionary presents approximately 1,500 words drawn from the content areas of the U.S. core curriculum in social studies, history, science, and math.

- There are eight thematic units, each divided into separate topics. Each topic has a full-page, color illustration on the right-hand page that places the words in context. The left-hand page features individual pictures taken from the illustration as a whole.

- $14.25

SparkChart on ESL Vocabulary
by Barnes and Noble, www.sparkcharts.com

- This set of charts is available online as a low-cost PDF downloadable file with several colorful pages of commonly used pictures and words.

- It is visually complex, but packed with functional pictures.

- $4.95

Topic Boards
by Millikin Communications Innovations, www. Communication-innovations.com

- There are topic boards of different sizes to support spoken communication that cover games, holidays, school topics, personal events, and stories.

- A sample script is included with each topic board to illustrate how to use the boards and to demonstrate the types of messages that can be conveyed using the boards.

- The cost is $5.00 to download specific topic boards. Durable backings are sold for $8.00.

Vidatak E-Z Board
by Vidatak, at www.vidatak.com

- The Vidatak E-Z Board (fourth generation) is an 11 × 17-inch preprinted dry-erase board.

- It is available in fifteen languages.

- $16.50

Computer Programs That Generate Text for Treatment

Several programs, that can be used to generate text for treatment, are available for purchase to assist the clinician in helping others improve verbal expression. Two programs are reviewed here because they relate directly to verbal expressive skills. Additional programs that can be used to generate treatment materials are discussed in Chapter 16, "Multi-Media Programs and Generating Printed Treatment Materials."

Title	Web Site	Price	PC	Mac	Online
SATPAC	www.satpac.com	$150.00	x		
Speech Tree	www.strokefamily.org	$129.95	x	x	x

SATPAC 4 (Systematic Articulation Training Program Accessing Computers)
by SATPAC Speech at www.satpac.com

- Lists can be printed for articulation therapy.

- The lists are generated with attention given to the use of facilitating contexts, coarticulation, and natural prosody. Numerous repetitions of the target sound are presented.

- A step-by-step protocol is provided for the articulation therapy process.

- There is an option of producing VCCV, CVCCV or VCCVC lists.

- Windows

- $150.00

Speech Tree
by Stroke Family at www.strokefamily.org

- Speech Tree is a Web-based program that features 3 levels and 16 different multi-sensory activities to begin to generate and speak in sentences.

- It includes over 400 words to make over 1000 sentences in 60 lessons.

- Users can print out the worksheets or use them on the computer.

- The user is shown words on a tree which can be used to form phrases. Common, practical and easy to choose words were selected.

- Target sentences are grouped into everyday themes such as food, people, and places.

- An assistant provides the verbal model and help while following the suggested activities in the manual.

- $129.95

Communication Devices With Voice

Many devices are available to assist users in the selection of multiple icons or words to convey complex ideas and concepts. Professionals need to keep in mind the client's level of acceptance, characteristics of the communication partners, the environment in which communication will take place, the features of the strategies and systems, and the capabilities and challenges of the client.

New devices are now combining the capabilities of speech-generating devices with Internet access and features of consumer electronics, such as cameras and cell phones. Some companies offer communication software that can be used on other computers (such as The Gus! Multimedia Speech System at www.gusinc.com), while others only offer their product along with the hardware.

Tips for Selecting a Communication Device

- It's important to decide the best way to represent language on the selected system: pictures, symbols, or words. Some clients with severe verbal apraxia have intact language skills and are able to use text to communicate. Those with severe aphasia are typically only able to use pictures and probably will have difficulty sequencing pictures to convey complex thoughts.

- You'll need to make clinical judgments about visual displays, sound output, and other software features.

- Consider the social network of the user, the environment, and the purposes for which the device will be used. A person with expressive communication deficits will communicate differently with family, close friends, paid caregivers, teachers, acquaintances, and strangers.

- Use expensive devices on a trial basis prior to purchase. Each state has an Assistive Technology Program. Many offer equipment loans at no cost. Many manufacturers rent their devices for trial use.

- Listen to the speech synthesizer used. The Microsoft voices and DECtalk synthesizers are more robotic-sounding than the AT&T voices, Acapela and NeoSpeech voices. You can buy the NeoSpeech, Acapela, RealSpeak and AT&T Voices at www.netxtup.com. They provide samples of the voices on the Web site. The voice files cost $25.00-$60.00 It is important to make sure the computer or device you want to use is compatible with the voice.

People Who Can Benefit From Augmentative Communication Devices

Detailed information about all of the devices on the market and their features is beyond the scope of this book. Many informative books and helpful Web sites are available, including, but not limited to the following:

- Augmentative and Alternative Communication for Adults With Acquired Neurologic Disorders, edited by David R. Beukelman, Kathryn M. Yorkston, and Joe Reichle ($44.95).

- Augmentative and Alternative Communication: Supporting Children and Adults With Complex Communication Needs, 3rd edition, by David R. Beukelman and Pat Mirenda ($69.95). Both are available at the following Web sites:
  - www.brookespublishing.com.
  - www.aacinstitute.org
  - www.aacpartners.com
  - www.abilityhub.com

- www.ablenetinc.com
- www.assistivetech.net
- www.ataccess.org
- www.closingthegap.com
- www.rehabtool.com
- www.ussaac.org
- www.woodlaketechnologies.com

Direct-Select, One-Level, Voice Output Communication Devices

These are relatively simple devices where messages are created on the device or are already programmed and activated by pressing a button to select a picture, word, or phrase. These direct-select, one-level, voice output communication devices include everything from talking picture frames and talking photo albums available at Radio Shack and Sharper Image to more specialized tools. Numerous alternatives are available from AbleNet, Enabling Devices, and Mayer-Johnson.

Direct-select, one-level, talking communication devices are great therapy tools for working on all language modalities and can be used as a stepping stone to determine readiness for more complex devices. These "talking" devices use pictures and words that the person who programs the device determines are most important for the client to communicate. When the user selects the picture, a prerecorded word or phrase is played aloud on the device. By selecting a picture or word, users may be able to "verbalize" basic needs and wants in real life and practice the utterances in therapy. If a client is unable to initiate use of these tools, the devices are often helpful for the communication partner. The combination of the picture and voice output helps comprehension. These talking devices are also helpful when a client is unable to rely on nonverbal communication (writing, gesturing, or drawing) for long-distance communication.

Title	Web Site	Price
Boardmaker Activity Pad	www.mayer-johnson.com	$795.00
GoTalk	www.attainmentcompany.com	$12.00 - $249.00
Listen to Me	Available at https://www.saltillo.com/shop	$79.00

Title	Web Site	Price
Talking Photo Albums	www.augcominc.com	$29.00
The AAC Idea Book: Creative Ways to Use Talking Photo Albums	www.augcominc.com	$45.00
The Children's Talking Dictionary with Spell Corrector	www.franklin.com	$59.95
Talking Language Master	www.franklin.com	$129.94 or $450.00 for the Special Edition version

Boardmaker Activity Pad
by Mayer-Johnson at www.mayer-johnson.com

- This device uses voice output, visual stimulation, and tactile activations.

- Printed activities are inserted into SmartPockets that slide into the device.

- Buttons are assigned and recorded and everything is saved to a chip on the Smart Pocket. Each pocket carries its own recording time.

- Free form layouts allow buttons to be located almost anywhere that they can be made switch accessible.

- Ten SmartPockets are included with at least 4 minutes of total recording time and up to 32 programmable buttons per side.

- Over 125 Boardmaker sample activities and templates are included.

- Windows and Mac

- $795.00 (an additional $200.00 includes the Boardmaker CD)

GoTalk
by Attainment Company, available at www.attainmentcompany.com

- Several versions are available, with varying numbers of pictures.

- Multiple layers of pictures can be recorded.

- The price range is from $12.00 for GoTalk One to $249.00 for GoTalk 20+.

Listen to Me
by DTK Enterprises, available at https://www.saltillo.com/shop

- This one-level communication device is accessed by pressing the keys on the front.

- The 12 keys have sleeves that allow graphics to be inserted onto the faces.

- $79.00

Talking Photo Albums
available at www.augcominc.com

- Talking photo albums enable the user to press a section on the bottom of an album page and hear spoken words corresponding to a picture made by the person who programmed it.

- The recordings can be of single words naming the picture or phrases describing the photo.

- $29.00

The AAC Idea Book: Creative Ways to Use Talking Photo Albums
by Sarah W. Blackstone and Harvey Pressman, www.augcominc.com

- This book contains twenty-one ideas contributed by fourteen AAC experts regarding the many ways to use a talking photo album in therapy.

- You can use the talking photo album to give instructions, tell stories, record autobiographical information, facilitate daily conversation, help order in restaurants, and facilitate memory.

- $45.00

The Children's Talking Dictionary With Spell Corrector
by Franklin Products, www.franklin.com

- This 40,000-word talking dictionary has easy-to-understand definitions and users can program personal word lists.

- Spelling correction verifies or corrects spelling.

- Missing letter search allows people to enter a question mark for missing letters to find words.

- This product speaks letters, words, and definitions.

- The Talking Dictionary with Spell Corrector is helpful for people who can start to type a word and then can use it to self-cue and read aloud or let the device say it aloud.

- $59.95

Talking Language Master
by Franklin Products, www.franklin.com

- This handheld dictionary offers full speech controls to read screens or speak individual words at selected speeds.

- Users can save words and messages.

- $129.94 or $450.00 for the special edition.

Dynamic, Dedicated, Communication Devices

Devices with dynamic display capabilities automatically change the picture displays and corresponding messages using internal hyperlinks. Novel messages can be communicated through sequential selection of pictures or words. Some of the devices are on tablet PCs with a touch screen, some are on smaller handheld computer units, and some are on dedicated laptops. Prices are available directly from the vendors. They use either digitized or synthesized speech, and are specifically designed to replace or augment speech. Digitized communication devices use recorded speech for the messages that will be heard by the communicators. Synthesized communication devices translate text into electronic speech. Clients with severe language-based deficits seldom use these devices effectively. Initiating communication is a major obstacle. Most often, the clients who use these devices for functional communication have more of a speech deficit such as dysarthria or apraxia rather than a language deficit such as aphasia. Medicare and other reimbursement services may pay for them given sufficient documentation.

Company	Web Site
DynaVox Technologies	www.dynavoxsys.com
Gus Communications	www.gusinc.com
Lingraphicare, Inc.	www.aphasia.com
Prentke Romich Company	www.prentrom.com
Saltillo Corporation	www.saltillo.com
Blink Twice	www.blink-twice.com
Words+	www.words-plus.com

DynaVox Technologies
available at www.dynavoxsys.com

- DynaVox brand dedicated speech-output devices include the DynaVox DV4, DynaVox MT4, MightyMo, MiniMo, DynaWrite, and Dynamo.

- The Impact line of communication devices includes the Tablet XL, the PalmTop, and the handheld Impact.

Gus Communications
available at www.gusinc.com

- Gus Communications offers a wide variety of Pocket PC and Windows-based speech (AAC) and computer access solutions such as The Pocket Communicator, The Communicator 2000, The Communicator Q1, and The Communicator 6,000.

- The software is designed specifically for adults with communication or physical disabilities.

The Lingraphica Express
by Lingraphicare, Inc., www.aphasia.com

- The Lingraphica Express 2 is a speech-generating device designed specifically for aphasia.

- It contains more than 6,000 words represented by icons which can be customized. The user chooses the icons to express his or her thoughts and needs, which the device then turns into spoken audible words or sentences. These can be saved for easy future access.

- The newest versions use a touch screen for direct selection.

- It includes hundreds of exercises to improve all many aspects of communication. An answer book is provided.

- A built-in patient evaluation provides a structured way to determine a patient's level and communication needs in one step.

- A built-in patient evaluation provides a structured way to determine a patient's level and communication needs in one step.

- It is available in Spanish.

Prentke Romich Company products (PRC)
available at www.prentrom.com

- PRC develops and manufactures many augmentative communication devices, computer access products, and other assistive technology products for people with severe disabilities.

- The Eco-14 is a new AAC aid and Windows XP-based compuer which became available in the Spring of 2007. Its AAC devices include the Pathfinder, Vanguard, Vantage, and SpringBoard.

- Prentke Romich uses Minspeak on the majority of its dedicated communication systems. This system helps the user with a combination of pre-stored vocabulary. The words that are representative of different parts of speech (verbs, nouns, articles, descriptors, etc) are presented together on a page based on the associated meanings of picture graphic symbols. Spelling and word prediction available.

Saltillo Corporation
available at www.saltillo.com

- Saltillo Corporation produces voice output, communication devices, as well as voice amplification and memory assistance products.

- They produce the ChatPC-M3 and ChatBox products.

Tango!
by Blink Twice, www.blink-twice.com

- Tango! is a device that comes with 2,500 prerecorded customizable phrases and newly designed symbols, as well as a built-in camera, video morphing capability, and flash.

- The user needs to be able to categorize items in order to find them.

- A pop-up keyboard and key phrase bank is always available.

- This device is designed primarily for children and teens to help them get up and running quickly.

- It features multiple scanning and mounting options.

Words+
available at www.words-plus.com

- Words+ develops several lines of communication systems, such as Say-It! SAM, TuffTalker, and Freedom Toughbook, and handheld communication devices such as MessageMates.

Dynamic Display, Communication Software

Several companies offer software that users can install on their own computers to turn them into communication devices. There is controversy in the professional world about this approach. On the positive side, users can then save the expense of purchasing another computer on which the dedicated communication devices are produced. When users purchase the communication software, they can use the computer they have with other software and features, such as Internet access and the use of word processing programs. A negative view is that the computer might not offer features that are needed for functional communication devices, such as "instant on" features, high-quality speakers, durability, and long battery life.

Title	Web Site	Price	PC	Mac	Other
Boardmaker with Speaking Dynamically Pro for Windows	www.mayer-johnson.com	$649.00	x		
DynaVox Speaking Software for Windows	www.dynavoxsys.com	$2,495.00	x		
EZ Keys XP	www.wordsplus.com	$1,395.00	x		
Gus! Easy Talk for Pocket PCs	www.gusinc.com	$295.00			Pocket PC
Gus! Easy Talk for Windows	www.gusinc.com	$295.00	x		
Gus! Multimedia Speech System for Windows	www.gusinc.com	$695.00	x		
Gus! Pocket Communicator	www.gusinc.com	$595.00			Pocket PC
Nextup Talker	www.talktome.com	$99.95	x		Tablet PC
Say it! Sam PC	www.wordsplus.com	$1,395.00	x		
Speech Pro	www.guscommunications.com	$895.00	x		

Boardmaker with Speaking Dynamically Pro Combo v6 for Windows
by Mayer-Johnson www.mayer-johnson.com

- Speaking Dynamically Pro is a dynamic screen communication program that turns the computer into a speech-output device and can be used to create educational interactive activities. It can play recorded (digitized) speech, speak text messages, open pop-up boards, link to other boards.

- Features include abbreviation expansion and word prediction to help build sentences with symbols or text.

- It Includes more than 4,500 PCS in both black-and-white and color, over 300 templates for schedules, device overlays, calendars, song boards, and 42 languages. It comes with assorted grids for communication boards or overlays.

- $649.00

DynaVox Speaking Software for Windows
available at www.dynavoxsys.com

- DynaVox Series 4 Speaking Software provides the communication software from its dedicated communication devices that can be used on a mainstream tablet, laptop, or desktop computer.

- It offers word, character, and recency prediction, abbreviation expansion, 17 pre-programmed page sets with 1200+ communication pages, multiple voice options, DynaSyms and Picture Communication Symbols, and timesaving communication and programming tools.

- This software can be purchased as companion software if the client already owns a DynaVox Dedicated Communication Device or as stand-alone software.

- Windows

- $2,495.00

EZ Keys XP
by Words+, www.wordsplus.com

- EZ Keys XP is designed for users who have at least a third-grade reading level and cannot speak, or for users who speak and desire adapted computer access.

- Thousands of phrases and sentences can be stored and rapidly retrieved using EZ Keys XP's Instant Phrases. Phrases can be grouped according to subject, such as family matters, sports, personal needs, jokes, or hobbies, and then use them quickly in everyday conversations.

- A variety of access modes, including standard keyboard, expanded keyboard, joystick, single-switch and multiple-switch scanning, and Morse code are available. A "no voice" version of EZ Keys XP is also available.

- Using a modem or fax/modem, you can send and receive messages or explore the World Wide Web.

- Windows

- $1,395.00

Gus! Easy Talk for Pocket PCs and Gus! Easy Talk for Windows
available at www.gusinc.com

- Phrases are categorized by topic. The user selects a topic and then the phrase to be spoken. He or she selects the Speak button to hear it.

- To string several phrases together, the user clicks the Append box and then selects as many phrases from different topics.

- $295.00

Gus! Multimedia Speech System for Windows
available at www.gusinc.com

- The Gus! Multimedia Speech System package includes a bundle of different communication and speech programs that include:

- Gus! Multimedia Speech System — dynamic display, communication software

- Gus! Talking Keyboard—talking word processor

- Gus! Easy Talk—conversational speech organized by topics and phrases

- Gus! Speak Clipboard—speaks the contents of the Windows clipboard

- Gus! Talking Calculator—on-screen calculator with speech output

- Gus! Symbol Set—communication symbol library containing over four thousand symbols

- Gus! Mouse—a switch-adapted mouse for switch/scanning users

- Windows

- $695.00

Gus! Pocket Communicator
available at www.gusinc.com

- This product is designed for people with communication or speech disorders who require a small, user-friendly, speech system and have the physical ability to use a handheld computer.

- It offers unlimited pages of words and phrases, along with the ability to create new words and phrases on the fly.

- Available as software only or bundled with a Pocket PC

- $595.00

NextUp Talker
by NextUp.com, www.talktome.com

- NextUp Talker is a Text To Speech application specifically designed for people who have lost their voices temporarily or permanently.

- It was developed to facilitate communication with fewer delays due to typing by using predefined, often used phrases and user created abbreviations.

- It adapts to the users style and speed with options to speak each word, sentence, or paragraph as they are typed, or on demand.

- The user can insert actual sound files along with speech.

- This software comes bundled with Mike and Crystal Natural Voices from AT&T or Kate and Paul from Neospeech.

- Windows or Tablet PC

- $99.95

Say it! Sam PC
by Words+, www.wordsplus.com

- This software uses a text and picture communication system that includes both a dynamic display interface and an intelligent keyboard interface.

- Quick and easy setup includes pre-designed pages.

- A variety of voices is available, including AT&T Natural Voices.

- Features such as phrase prediction, abbreviation expansion and an auto-learning feature that learns the vocabulary that is used facilitate rapid communication.

- There are environmental control features for lights, TV, DVD player and more with the optional U-Control III environmental control.

- This program can be used as part of a complete Words+ Communication system, or ready to install on a tablet, laptop, or desktop computer.

- Windows

- $1,395.00

Speech Pro
by Gus Communications, www.gusinc.com

- This program is switch scanning accessible

- There are 4 main areas:

- Top Area — Text-to-speech window with word prediction

- Keyboard Area — On-screen keyboard for touch screen, mouse, or other pointing device

- Words Area — 100 most commonly used English words. Can be arranged in any configuration, or removed.

- Tab Area (bottom) — "Dynamic display" features. Choose a tab and only the words area changes to the selected word category (e.g., People). Allows dynamic page links to unlimited words templates.

- Each button can contain text of any length.

- It is compatible with speech synthesizers in any language.

- Windows XP or Vista

Devices and Software Using a Client's Own Speech To Clarify the Message

Several devices and software programs make residual verbal expression abilities more functional.

Voice amplifiers and a product that clarifies the speech called the Voice Enhancer are helpful for people with Parkinson's, MS, and other conditions that cause a strain on the larynx. They also are helpful for professionals who place heavy demands on their voices such as teachers, trainers, and presenters. Clients with benign lesions like nodules resulting from vocal abuse such as yelling, screaming, loud talking, or singing can also benefit from amplifiers and clarifiers. The devices offer hands-free communication and are lightweight. They can be worn on a belt, in a pocket, or around the neck. Medicare covers amplifiers for some people.

Title	Web Site	Price
ChatterVox	www.chattervox.com	$249.00
Speech Enhancer	www.speechenhancer.com	N/A
Voice Saver	www.maxiaids.com www.hearmore.com www.soundbytes.com	$119.95
SentenceShaper	www.speechenhancer.com	$249.00

ChatterVox
by ChatterVox at www.chattervox.com and also sold at www.enablemart.com

- This voice amplification system gives fifteen decibels of voice boost.

- It is a lightweight unit that is designed to be worn at the waist.

- There are both over-the-ear and collar-style microphones. Both have an adjustable boom, so that the microphone can be positioned very close to the mouth for the best amplification with the least vocal effort.

- $249.00

Speech Enhancer
by Voicewave Technology, www.speechenhancer.com

- This device makes speech clearer, restores an inaudible voice, and boosts computer speech-recognition accuracy.

- Each system has a microphone and a lightweight voice-processing unit that is worn at the waist or mounted on a wheelchair.

- Various models offer telephone and wireless capabilities and support for computer speech-recognition software.

- It is available only through an evaluation by an independent certified evaluator who provides the pricing information.

Voice Saver
by Califone, sold at www.maxiaides.com, www.hearmore.com, and www.soundbytes.com,

- Two-watt amplifier with separate tone and volume controls.

- Plug in the microphone, clip it to your belt, and turn it on.

- It weighs less than a pound and comes complete with a headset microphone, four AA rechargeable batteries, a charging adaptor, and an adjustable belt.

- $119.95

The following sites provide additional products and information:

- www.luminaud.com
- www.radioshack.com
- www.saltillo.com
- www.speechaid.com
- www.communicativemedical.com
- www.soundbytes.com
- www.closedloopcommunications.com

SentenceShaper
by Psycholinguistic Technologies at www.sentenceshaper.com

- This program helps people with significant aphasia and verbal apraxia by recording parts of intelligible speech and allowing the user to produce narratives by selecting them to communicate messages.

- The purpose of SentenceShaper is to facilitate spoken language by serving as a "processing prosthesis." It allows users to record spoken fragments and assemble them into sentences by manipulating icons on a computer screen.

- Windows

- $195.00

Emergency Alerts, Telephones, Videophones and Assistive Options

Emergency Alerts

For people who are alone, a subscription to a medical alert service that is connected to a local hospital can be helpful. For more information, go to one of the following Web sites:

- www.vital-linkinc.com

- www.LifelineSystems.com

- www.seniorservices.org

The telephone is one of the main tools of our everyday lives. It is an important means of communicating in emergencies, accessing information, and maintaining contact with family and friends. Yet, it is difficult to use for people with verbal expression issues. Without its benefits, depression and feelings of isolation can become problematic and hinder the rehabilitation and learning process. We can help clients compensate for phone-related challenges in many ways.

Relay Phone Assistance

A telecommunications relay service is provided free of charge to anyone who needs communication assistance. For more information about this, contact www.fcc.gov/cgb/dro/trs.html.

- Speech-to-speech (STS) service is for a person with a speech disability. The individual talks to a communications assistant with special training in listening and understanding a variety of speech disorders. The communications assistant repeats everything, making the caller's words clear and understandable, and then makes the call for that person.

- In hearing carryover (HCO)—so called because the person with the speech disability can hear the other party's voice—people who have difficulty speaking on the phone can place or receive calls by typing what they want to say using a special telephone called a text telephone (TTY). A communications assistant then reads their words to the person they called. Three-way calling is necessary for an HCO call.

- The FCC has reserved 711 for relay service access. Just as 411 can be called for information, 711 can be dialed to connect to relay service anywhere in the United States.

Cell Phones

Cell phones have become increasingly important in today's society. Pay phones are rare and often do not function. People with difficulty communicating should carry a cell phone if they travel alone in the community, so that they can call others who are familiar with their situation for help as needed.

For clients who have relatively preserved cognitive abilities, sequencing skills, and manual dexterity, features of smart phones can augment communication abilities. Phones now come equipped with cameras, text messaging, Web access, and PDAs (personal digital assistants). With a bit of imagination and creativity, these devices can become powerful communication assistants. The following useful features provide examples:

- Address book — helpful for recalling names of people
- Calendar — helpful for remembering and organizing and for referring to names, dates, and places in conversation
- Still and video cameras — provide an effective way to communicate by sending a person a picture of a situation, a person, a place, or an event

In addition, quite a few software programs are compatible with Pocket PCs, Palm-based handhelds, and phones and can assist with communication. Some are picture-based, and others are text-based. Many have the same features as dedicated communication devices. More information can be found at these Web sites:

Title	Web Site	Price
Gus! Communicator	www.gusinc.com	$1,995.00
Mobile Communication Suite	www.ablelinktech.com	$899.00

Gus! Communicator X700
by Gus Communications, www.gusinc.com

- This device includes Treo Smartphone 700w and Gus speech software, a Pocket PC, cell phone, camera, and speech device, with high-speed Internet access.

- $1,995.00

Mobile Communication Suite
by AbleLink Technologies, www.ablelinktech.com

- The main purpose of this suite is to make calls at predetermined time intervals. If the cue is to make a phone call, then the accessible phone application launches and the user can complete the cell call.

- Caregivers set up the various daily, weekly, and monthly tasks and time cues with audio and custom pictures on the computer.

- The Pocket PC phone allows the use of an accessible cell phone while combining the benefits of AbleLink's scheduling application. This can remind the user to make a phone call at a preset time, maintaining the benefits of the Pocket PC platform.

- The Mobile Communications Suite comes ready to go with a custom Pocket PC phone, Pocket ACE (Accessible Communication Enabler phone application), Schedule Assistant (custom audio-visual cuing), and Discovery Desktop (a custom Windows desktop).

- $899.00

Adapted Cell Phones

People with physical, communication, or cognitive disabilities frequently find the use of a standard handset with small buttons difficult to use. A few phones like these below may help.

Title	Web Site	Price
Firefly	www.fireflymobile.com	$79.99
TalkingAide Wireless	www.zygo-usa.com	$5,995.00
SafeGuardian	www.safeguardian.com	$299.95

Firefly
from Firefly Mobile, www.fireflymobile.com

- This phone features two big buttons that can be programmed to dial numbers, which makes it easy to use. It is colorful with flashing lights.

- It is designed for children, but helpful for all ages.

- $79.99

TalkingAide Wireless
by Zygo Industries at www.zygo-usa.com

- The TalkingAide Wireless is a text-to-speech device designed specifically for cell phone and e-mail use. It uses DECtalk speech synthesis with seven voices.

- There is a typing mode (up to 20,000 characters) and a chat mode for writing and engaging in secondary conversations.

- Function keys can be used easy selection of onscreen options such as word completion predictions.

- There is a 6" display with backlighting and 3 font sizes. It weighs 3.5 pounds, has a handle, and is 10.5x8.75x3 inches.

- $5,995.00

SafeGuardian
by Clayton Communications, www.safeguardian.com

- This is an emergency-only phone with a big, red 911 button. The user can call and speak with a live personal assistant simply by pressing the Call button.

- The phone includes a 95-decibel alarm to attract help in an emergency. It also has a GPS (Global Positioning System) locator.

- $299.95

Adapted Landline Phones

Large buttons, preprogrammed numbers, pictures for preprogrammed locations or people, and integrated answering machines are helpful phone features for people with challenges.

Title	Web Site	Price
Dialogue VCO Phone	Available at www.enablemart.com www.potomactech.com www.lifewithease.com	Approx. $149.95

Title	Web Site	Price
Pocket VCO	www.turningpointtechnology.com www.enablemart.com	Approx. $199.95
P-300 Photo Phone	www.enablemart.com 101phones.com	$59.95
Compact/C Portable TTY	101phones.com www.enablemart.com www.hearmore.com	$299.00
LinkCLASSIC	www.assistivetech.com	$2,495.00

Dialogue VCO Phone

by Ameriphone, available at www.enablemart.com, www.potomactech.com

- This is a read-and-talk telephone.

- The user reads responses on the display screen and speaks into the handset.

- Calls must be placed through the toll-free relay service by calling 711.

- Features include 30x amplification, programmable memory, and emergency buttons.

- $149.95

Pocket VCO

available at www.enablemart.com

- The Pocket Speak and Read VCO with Direct Connect provides the ability to attach to any TTY-compatible cell phone, pay phone, cordless phone, or traditional phone or call box.

- $199.95

Photo Phone

available at www.101phones.com

- This phone features nine locations where pictures can be placed.

- The user touches the photo and the number is automatically speed dialed.

- It has easy-to-see, oversized keypad buttons. The ringing volume can go up to ten times the standard sound level.

- The handset is hearing aid, T-coil compatible. There is also a bright visual ring flasher. $59.95

Compact/C Portable TTY
available at www.hearmore.com

- This full-featured TTY is very small and can connect with a compatible cell phone or any public phone.
- The 32K memory stores TTY conversations, memos, and important phone numbers.
- There is a two-line display.
- $299.00

LinkCLASSIC
from Assistive Technologies at www.assistivetech.com

- This phone has a full-sized keyboard that speaks as you type or scan.
- Key words and phrases can be retrieved and spoken instantly.
- It has word prediction and single-switch scanning, as well as a choice of nine voices and six languages.
- The Link has a built-in telephone with on-screen dialer, the ability to upload and store files to a computer, and adjustable volume, pitch, and rate. It weighs 2.2 pounds.
- $2,495.00

Videophones

Telephones that can transmit and receive both video and audio signals, allowing people to see as well as hear each other, are called videophones. They have become much more affordable and make distance communication easier. Some videophones resemble regular phones with the use of video. Face-to-face contact is very helpful for people with communication deficits. The use of gesture, facial expression, contextual cues, calendars, writing, and communication devices to augment verbal utterances helps with the effectiveness of the interaction. Being able to see the person you are talking to is a big advantage.

For several options, go to these Web sites:

- www.videophonesales.com
- www.videophoneconnection.com

There are also videophones that are Internet-based and require the use of a computer with a Web cam. An example is Skype at www.skype.com. Skype is a program for making free calls over the Internet to anyone who also has Skype. It's free and easy to download and use, and it works with most computers. Web cameras on either end enable the speakers to see the other party. The calls have excellent sound quality and are highly secure, with end-to-end encryption.

Music

Music can add a new dimension to therapy sessions. A very effective tool, it is often overlooked in the development and remediation of speech and language — especially for people with significant verbal apraxia or dysfluency.

- The Internet provides a wide array of recorded music. The two most popular sites are iTunes.com and Napster.com. You can purchase songs for ninety-nine cents, and listen to short clips for free. Many of the accompanying lyrics can be printed from www.azlyrics.com

- It is helpful to encourage family members to play familiar repetitive music.

- Incorporate playing instruments such as the piano into sessions if instrumental music has been an important part of a client's life.

- In certain cases, it is helpful to develop a working relationship with a music therapist to promote combined efforts to reach verbal expression goals. More information about music therapists can be found at www.musictherapy.org.

Here are a few products that help clinicians use music to improve verbal expression skills.

CHAT
by Aphasia Therapy Products, www.aphasia-therapy.com

- A section of the CHAT software uses musical notes on a treble clef with melodic repetition of functional words and phrases—with and without text.

- Windows

- $169.50

R in the Car
by Alida Engel at www.speech-therapy-products.com

- Ten fun songs are included on an audio CD to practice the "R" sound.

- $19.95

Sing-Along with ElderSong
available at www.eldersong.com

- Familiar songs are a great way to tap into the right side of the brain to help with verbal expression.

- ElderSong offers a wide variety of sing-along CDs that include well-known songs and large-print lyric books.

- Approximately $14.95.

Companies at the following Web sites offer music-based products to use with children for speech development:

- Precision Songs at www.precisionsongs.com

- Good Foundations at www.goodfoundations.net

- Speechville Express at www.speechville.com

- Kids' Express Train at www.expresstrain.org

- Institute of Applied Psychomusicology at www.soundpsych.com

Training Communication Partners

In addition to working directly with the people who have communication deficits, it is very important to work with those with whom they will spend most of their time communicating. Parents, spouses, children, specialists, and teachers will typically benefit from assistance acquiring the necessary strategies, skills, and approach to use to facilitate effective communication.

For additional information on this topic check out:

- www.paulakluth.com/articles/commpartner.html

- www.communicationmatters.org.uk/Publications/Focus_On/FO_How_to_be_a _Good_Listener/fo_how_to_be_a_good_listener.html

Chapter 11:
Treatment and Technology To Improve Auditory Comprehension

It is devastating when a person is unable to understand spoken language. Listening and understanding play a crucial role in our daily lives. In conversation, we translate speech into meaningful language. As we listen, we decode and identify meaningful words effortlessly.

In many ways, computers and technology can help adults and children who have a hard time understanding what is said to them. Computers can both compensate for and provide drill and practice for activities to improve the comprehension of words, directions, and conversations. Computer use empowers the client to increase the time spent practicing skills taught by the communication and cognitive specialist.

People with auditory comprehension and processing deficits may have the following characteristics:

- Demonstrate a short attention span

- Show signs of distractibility

- Display an oversensitivity to sounds

- Misinterpret what is said to them

- Confuse words

- Need frequent repetition

- Be unable to follow directions

- Have difficulty with speech and verbal expression

- Show poor reading comprehension

In children, a central auditory processing disorder (CAPD) occurs when the ear and the brain do not coordinate fully. Auditory information breaks down somewhere beyond the ear.

In adults, language-based, auditory comprehension deficits are referred to as "receptive aphasia." The causes are varied and they can include head trauma and stroke.

As with other language modalities, working to improve auditory comprehension is a complex task. The reasons for the difficulty need to be thoroughly evaluated, so that the strategies and practice during therapy are appropriate. A person may appear not to understand, but the problem may be complicated by a variety of other issues, such as problems with hearing, processing, and memory. This guide does not replace formal professional training in evaluation and treatment. Its purpose is to provide a wide variety of tools for professionals who help people with communication and cognitive challenges.

Therapy Approach

When helping people who have difficulty understanding what is said to them, it is helpful to find other ways to enhance the message being said.

- Show communication partners how to use the environment to support the message. The use of gestures, pictures, written words, calendars, clocks, objects, and actions can be used to facilitate communication.

- Speak more slowly, face the listener, and articulate speech well to facilitate comprehension.

- Minimize external distractions such as the TV and other extraneous visual and auditory stimuli.

- Provide multi-sensory cues to assist with comprehension. Clients do best when they can see a word, hear a word, and perhaps touch an object.

- Presenting words in their natural context improves comprehension. For instance, try to talk about food items while in the kitchen, or have a calendar to refer to while talking about dates.

Drill-and-Practice Software

Many software programs can help improve auditory comprehension skills. In addition to the auditory-focused software presented in this chapter, a review of the software for clients with verbal expression, reading comprehension and memory deficits is suggested; many of those are also helpful with auditory comprehension disabilities. Programs listed in this chapter may also be helpful toward improving other areas of communication and cognition.

Title	Web Site	Price	PC	Mac	Other
Direction Following Out Loud+ (verbal and written)	www.bungalowsoftware.com	$189.50	x		
Earobics	www.earobics.com	$299.00	x		

Title	Web Site	Price	PC	Mac	Other
Fast ForWord	www.fastforword.com	Language software $900.00	x	x	
Following Directions: One and Two-Level Commands	www.laureatelearning.com	$175.00	x	x	
My House, My Town, and My School: The Language Activities of Daily Living Series	www.laureatelearning	Each $150.00	x	x	
No-Glamour Auditory Processing	www.linguisystems.com	$41.95	x	x	
Parrot Software	www.parrotsoftware.com	Per month $24.95	x		x
English (U.S.) Level 1	www.rosettastone.com	CD $195.00 Per month online $49.95	x	x	x
The Listening Program	www.advancedbrain.com	$399.95			CD player with head-phones
Understanding Questions Out Loud	www.bungalowsoftware.com	$189.50	x		

Direction Following Out Loud+ (verbal and written)
by Bungalow Software, www.bungalowsoftware.com

- The user hears and/or reads directions and follows them by moving shapes on the screen with the mouse or keyboard.

- If the incorrect answer is given, the program provides helpful suggestions in a human voice.

- Task complexity can be controlled. When working with high-level clients, it may be helpful to adapt the task and have the client practice writing notes from lengthy spoken directions prior to task completion to assist with accurate retention of the information.

- $189.50

Earobics
by Cognitive Concepts, www.earobics.com

- This program uses a game-style format that includes six interactive programs with over three hundred levels of multimedia instruction to help improve reading, spelling, and comprehension.

- It uses adaptive training, acoustic enhancement of the speech signal, and systematic control of key learning variables. The adaptive training technology automatically adjusts game play to the skill level and progress of each user. It systematically controls the amount of visual cueing and auditory feedback, the rate at which sounds are presented, the length of sound units, and the amount of background noise.

- The games develop attention and memory. Earobics offers automatic goal writing in IEP format and performance charting.

- This program is available online or on a CD.

- Windows

- The Earobics program for professionals costs $299.00.

- The cost for families is $45.00

Fast ForWord
by Scientific Learning Corporation, www.fastforword.com

- Fast ForWord language software builds the cognitive skills of memory, attention, processing, and sequencing in the context of key language and reading skills. This includes listening accuracy, phonological awareness, and language structures.

- Supplemental and companion software are available on the Web site.

- Providers are required to take a free online training course, which usually takes about five hours.

- A single-user license for the language software is $900.00.

Following Directions: One and Two-Level Commands
by Laureate Learning Systems, www.laureatelearning.com

- This program offers twenty-four different activities that teach one-level, sequential, and two-level commands using spatial relations and directional terms.

- Windows and Mac

- $175.00

My House, My Town, and My School: The Language Activities of Daily Living Series
by Laureate Learning Systems, www.laureatelearning.com

- Several options to customize the lessons are offered. There are six scenes in each program.

- In the Identify Names section, the user selects the item named.

- In the Identify Functions/Descriptions tasks, the user finds a described item.

- Windows and Mac

- $150.00 each

No-Glamour Auditory Processing Interactive Software
by Carolyn LoGiudice, www.linguisystems.com

- Includes simple, auditory reception skills to complex, problem-solving tasks.

- There are 400 items, arranged in order of complexity, allow for mastery of nine auditory processing skills necessary for academic success: auditory reception, absurdities, details, main idea, phonological awareness, following directions, comprehension, exclusion, problem solving and riddles.

- Windows or Mac

- $41.95

Parrot Software
available at www.parrotsoftware.com

- This online subscription offers many programs (list follows) that focus on attention and memory. The subscription includes seventy different rehabilitation programs. It is Windows compatible and $24.95 a month for the online subscription.

- Auditory and Visual Instructions — Four geometric forms are displayed. A description of one of the geometric forms is presented using the attributes of size, color, and shape (e.g., large, yellow, square). The user must identify the geometric form that fits the description.

- Listening Skills — A random selection of verbal instructions with one to five critical elements is presented, and the user must follow the instructions. The tasks consist of assigning colors to specific geometric forms displayed on the screen.

- Memory for Directions — Written or spoken directions are given requesting that small pictures be moved to special locations on the screen with a mouse.

English (U.S.) Level 1
by Rosetta Stone at www.rosettastone.com

- Level 1 includes over 3,500 real-life images and phrases in ninety-two lessons. It is available in 29 languages.

- This program enables the user to specify the modality targeted. If the icon of the speaker is selected, the tasks are auditory.

- Windows and Mac

- $195.00 for the CD or $49.95 for a one-month online subscription

The Listening Program
by Advanced Brain Technologies, www.advancedbrain.com

- The Listening Program is a music-based auditory stimulation method that trains the brain to improve the auditory skills needed to listen, learn, and communicate.

- The program consists of fifteen to thirty minutes a day of music specifically recorded for this purpose.

- $399.95 The price includes a phone consultation and progress follow up. Professional training is needed to become a provider.

Understanding Questions Out Loud
by Bungalow Software, www.bungalowsoftware.com

- This program provides practice with understanding various types of questions: Who? What? When? Where? Why? and How?

- The type and number of questions asked can be tailored to the needs of the user. Information can be presented auditorally as well as visually.

- Windows

- $189.50

Long-Distance Communication

Communicating on the phone is difficult if someone has a hard time with auditory comprehension. Several solutions are available.

Telephones

Special landlines, cell phones, videophones, and relay services can help people with auditory comprehension deficits communicate over a distance. There are many types. Please refer to Chapter 10, "Additional Tools and Resources To Improve Verbal Expression," for more information on adapted telephones.

Text

For a person who has difficulty understanding spoken language, text-based communication methods can augment comprehension. E-mailing, faxing, and instant messaging may be more effective when a client is attempting to communicate with someone who is not in his or her immediate environment.

Assistive Listening Devices

Assistive listening devices (ALDs) include a large variety of devices designed to improve comprehension in specific listening situations. Some are designed to be used with cochlear implants or hearing aids with a T-switch, while others are designed to be used alone. Assistive listening devices improve the listener's ability to hear by making the desired sound stand out from the background noise. Being able to hear can have a major impact on a person's ability to participate in social, academic, and work situations.

Additional information can be found on these Web sites:

- www.advancedhearing.com
- www.alds.com
- www.harriscomm.com
- www.hearinglossweb.com

Captioning

Closed Captioning

Closed captions contain text that is hidden within normal television broadcasts and on videotapes and DVDs. A television with the built-in caption decoder chip or an external decoder is needed to make the captions visible. It can typically be turned on or off by viewing the menu of options available with the TV. There's no special service to subscribe to in order to receive the captions. Captioning is made free for all viewers by the television and home video industries, and with the support of grants and donations. This multi-sensory experience of watching captioned TV has been shown to improve significantly the reading skills of children. In addition, people learning English can improve their language and vocabulary skills, and adults with auditory comprehension deficits can improve their comprehension of the spoken material.

Real-Time Captioning

Real-time captioning currently takes place when a person types what is said into a stenotype machine. The machine is connected to a computer with software that translates the shorthand into words in caption formats and standard spellings. It is now becoming possible to tape lectures and presentations, then to use voice recognition software to transcribe what is said. As technology advances, this procedure has enormous potential for helping people with communication and cognitive deficits. However, the accuracy of voice recognition software with dictation is inconsistent. Freeware for closed captioning may be found at http://ncam.wgbh.org/webaccess/magpie/.

Caption Mic Classroom
by Ultech, www.ultech.com

- Caption Mic ("Mic" as in "microphone") is a "do-it-yourself" captioning system that produces captions with the help of speech recognition technology. A voice captioner echoes what is spoken at an event, and the resulting captions are displayed on a TV monitor.
- $4,995.00

More information about captioning may be found at:

- www.ncicap.org
- www.mcpo.org
- www.robson.org

Chapter 12:
Treatment and Technology To Improve Reading Comprehension

Millions of people of all ages have difficulty reading. The deficits may be developmental or acquired. Impaired reading ability can be the result of a stroke, head injury, learning disability, cognitive deficit, or visual and perceptual problem. Some people have difficulty reading English because it's not their primary language. Deficits range in severity and the impact that they have on a person's life. Many people who are able to read may read slowly and have difficulty processing what they read. They may be able to understand the words in the text, but be unable to synthesize the information in order to find the main idea, identify implied information, paraphrase the content, locate desired information, or write about what they read.

Reading is a complex task. To help people effectively who are having difficulty reading, you need to understand where the problems arise. Reading issues can stem from auditory perception difficulties, visual perception difficulties, or language processing difficulties. The tools needed to improve and compensate for reading challenges of different etiologies vary. Successful use of assistive devices and drill-and-practice software depends on two factors: pairing the appropriate tools with the individual based on his or her deficits and training the individual to use them in everyday life.

People who have difficulty with reading may present with many different scenarios. They may have the following difficulties:

- Be able to read aloud well, but show poor comprehension.

- Understand the content, but not be able to remember it.

- Go thru the process of "reading" the newspaper each morning, but, when tested, show little comprehension of what they appeared to read.

- Get visually lost on the page or be unable to see the words.

- Show slow processing time, which makes it difficult to keep up with reading demands at school or work, or may prevent adults from reading for pleasure.

- Demonstrate the ability to read basic information, but be unable to process complex material.

- Have overall poor literacy skills.

- Speak another language.

Multi-Disciplinary Approach

It's often in the best interest of the client for professionals to initiate a multidisciplinary approach toward reading training and remediation.

- Make sure that people with reading challenges who are suspected of having visually based deficits be evaluated and treated by an ophthalmologist or neuro-ophthalmologist.

- Many professionals are able to assist in the treatment of reading challenges. Speech-language pathologists, occupational therapists, reading specialists, special education teachers, and vision specialists are trained to work on particular approaches to improve reading.

- If the client is a student, the Individuals with Disabilities Education Act requires that school personnel, in conjunction with the child's parents, develop an Individualized Education Program (IEP) for each student with learning disabilities who is eligible for special education.

- If the client is a person returning to work, the Americans with Disabilities Act (ADA) (www.usdoj.gov/crt/ada/adahom1.htm) requires that all employers provide reasonable accommodations for employees who are identified as having a disability.

There is quite a bit of current research concerning the potential causes of reading difficulties and the most effective treatment options. It's been proven that people who have difficulty reading have a better chance of comprehending and retaining the content of written material with a guided reading approach and if they can simultaneously see the words and hear them read aloud.

These are some helpful online resources:

- The International Reading Association, www.reading.org
- www.LDonline.org
- The National Institutes of Health, www.nichd.nih.gov/crmc/cdb/reading.htm
- The National Center for Technology Innovation offers a "Reading Matrix" at http://www.nationaltechcenter.org/matrix/default.asp. This feature provides a comparison of software for six reading purposes: Building Skills and Comprehension, Converting Text to Speech, Providing Text in Alternate Formats, Providing Electronic Resources, Organizing Ideas, and Integrating Literacy/Supports.

There are many treatment options to consider for both compensation and remediation of reading. In this chapter, the following topics are discussed:

- Software features

- Software to improve language-based reading comprehension deficits
- Software for vision-based reading deficits
- Computer accommodations for people with visual-perceptual deficits
- Assistive reading technology
- Text-to-speech
- Optical character recognition
- Alternative book formats
- Non-tech resources to help in reading treatment
- Additional resources to help improve reading

As with other goal areas, the computer offers clients a way to increase their time spent practicing skills learned in treatment sessions. Much of the software that is used to improve reading can also be used to improve written expression and memory. Different software programs offer different approaches and features to improve reading. They vary widely in price and targeted outcomes. Many allow clients and clinicians to experiment with customizing options to maximize their effectiveness in education and rehabilitation.

Software Features

During the software selection process, consider which of the following software features would be helpful for the client. These features may include the following abilities:

- To focus on the development of improved auditory-perceptual skills and phonics to assist with reading
- To pair text with graphics for users who can interpret pictures, but not the printed word
- To provide written material and drill and practice with effective strategies to facilitate comprehension and analysis
- To read aloud text that is printed on the computer screen, while also enlarging and highlighting the text
- To change the format of the text to make it easier to view
- To convert printed text from a paper or book into editable text to help with studying, to enable the material to be read aloud on a computer, or to be converted to WAV files for use in an MP3 or CD player
- To work on visual tracking and scanning to improve reading fluency
- To give pronunciations aloud and definitions for words using portable spell checkers, translators, and reading pens

Software for Language-Based Reading Comprehension Deficits

This section reviews software that offers a drill-and-practice approach to improve reading skills.

Most of these programs

- offer tasks at a variety of reading levels,
- can be customized,
- provide immediate feedback regarding the accuracy of the response, and
- document performance.

Keep in mind that new versions of software are frequently being released and features are being changed. It is important to review Web sites for more up-to-date and in-depth analysis of product comparisons.

Title	Web Site	Price	PC	Mac	Other
ACHIEVE! Phonics, Reading & Writing Grades 1-3	www.learningcompany.com	$19.99	x		
ACHIEVE! Writing and Language Arts Grades 3-6	www.learningcompany.com	$19.99	x		
Aphasia Tutor 1+: Words	www.bungalowsoftware.com	$199.00	x		
Aphasia Tutor 2+: Sentences Out Loud	www.bungalowsoftware.com	$199.00	x		
Aphasia Tutor 3: Story Reading	www.bungalowsoftware.com	$169.50	x		
Aphasia Tutor 4: Functional Reading	www.bungalowsoftware.com	$119.50	x		
Bailey's Book House	www.learningcompany.com	$59.95	x	x	
ClozePro	www.cricksoft.com	$199.00	x	x	

Title	Web Site	Price	PC	Mac	Other
Edmark Reading Program- Software Version	www.enablemart.com www.superduperinc.com	$475.00	x	x	
English (U.S.) Level 1	www.rosettastone.com	$195.00 Per month online $49.95	x	x	Online subscription
Fast ForWord	www.fastforword.com	$900.00	x	x	
Lexia Reading Software	www.lexialearning.com	Strategies for Older Students v4.0F, Family Edition $159.00	x	x	
Reading Comprehension Booster	www.meritsoftware.com	Home version $39.00	x		
Developing Critical Thinking Skills for Effective Reading	www.meritsoftware.com	Home version $39.00	x		
My House, My Town, and My School: The Language Activities of Daily Living Series	www.laureatelearning.com	Each $150.00	x	x	
On Track Reading Series	www.toolfactory.com	5-CD set $299.95	x	x	
Parrot Software Version 8.1	www.parrotsoftware.com	Per month online $24.95	x		Online subscription
Reader Rabbit Reading Learning System 2007	www.learningcompany.com	$19.99	x	x	
Reading Detective	www.criticalthinking.com	$64.99	x	x	

Title	Web Site	Price	PC	Mac	Other
Software					
Simon S.I.O	www.donjohnston.com	$149.00	x	x	
Thinking Reader	www.tomsnyder.com	$250.00	x	x	
Time4Learning	www.time4learning.com	$19.95 per month	X	X	Online
Understanding Questions Out Loud	www.bungalowsoftware.com	$149.50	X		
WordMaker	www.donjohnston.com	$149.00	x	x	

ACHIEVE! Phonics, Reading & Writing Grades 1-3
by The Learning Company, www.learningcompany.com

- Four programs are included:
    - Let's Go Read! I: An Island Adventure
    - Let's Go Read!2: An Ocean Adventure
    - Bailey's Book House
    - Stories and More: Time & Place
- Windows
- $19.99

ACHIEVE! Writing and Language Arts Grades 3-6
by The Learning Company, www.learningcompany.com

- The following four programs are included:
    - Word Munchers Deluxe
    - Schoolhouse Rock
    - The Writing Trek
    - Strategy Challenges Collection 2: In the Wild
- Windows
- $19.99

Aphasia Tutor 1+: Words Out Loud and Aphasia Tutor 2+: Sentences Out Loud
by Bungalow Software, www.bungalowsoftware.com

- The initial menu offers a variety of lessons in a multiple-choice format.

- The exercises progress in difficulty from words to phrases and then to sentence-level reading comprehension tasks.

- Depending on the selected level, exercises provide text and/or pictures.

- Text can be read aloud as needed for support.

- The text is large and the program is easy to use for people with severe deficits.

- Windows

- $199.00 per program

Aphasia Tutor 3: Story Reading
by Bungalow Software, www.bungalowsoftware.com

- This program improves reading comprehension at the paragraph and story levels.

- Lessons gradually increase in passage length and question complexity (including factual and inferential questions).

- The Reading Cursor highlights one word at a time to make reading easier.

- When errors are made, the program highlights where the appropriate answer can be found in the text.

- Windows

- $169.50 for the professional version

Aphasia Tutor 4: Functional Reading
by Bungalow Software, www.bungalowsoftware.com

- This software provides realistic reading materials such as medicine labels, want ads, and television guides.

- There are six levels for each section.

- Audiovisual feedback is provided to the user as needed.

- Windows

- $119.50 for the professional version

Bailey's Book House v4
by The Learning Company, www.learningcompany.com

- This program was designed for children who are in preschool through second grade.

- Children build a reading and writing foundation by exploring letters, words, rhyming, and sentence building.

- There are multimedia resources through graphic and spoken instruction, talking words, Discover modes, and Question & Answer modes.

- Greeting cards and storybooks can be printed.

- In this very engaging program they learn the following language features:

    - Discover letter names and sounds.

    - Learn uppercase and lowercase letters.

    - Study positional words, contextual clues, and sentence building.

    - Learn how to use common adjectives and prepositions.

    - Increase reading vocabulary.

    - Recognize consonant blends and form compound words.

    - Practice skills in word recognition, phonics, comprehension, phonemic awareness, written expression, vocabulary development, and word building.

    - Work through 10 questions in each of the nine activities: Elmo & Houdini, Letter Machine, Make-a-Story, Three-Letter Carnival, Read-A-Rhyme, Kid Cards, My Friend, Silly Songs, and Compound Hound.

- Windows or Mac

- $59.95

ClozePro
by Crick Software, www.cricksoft.com

- The clinician selects a body of text that can be either typed or copied from a Web site, an e-mail, or a document.

- They then choose words to remove from the text.

- Categories of words, such as verbs, nouns, or every fourth word, can be omitted.

- The missing words can be given in a grid at the bottom of the page or in a multiple-choice format.

- The user then selects words to place back into the text.

- This program offers customizable interfaces and detailed reporting capability to track progress, and it is fully switch-accessible.

- Many free downloadable activities that can be used with this software are available at www.learninggrids.com.

- Windows and Mac

- $199.00

Edmark Reading Program- Software Version
by Edmark available at www.enablemart.com and www.superduperinc.com in addition to other resellers.

- Using a whole word approach, this program teaches recognition and comprehension of words with built-in instructions, audio cues, and feedback.

- There are 29 multi-page stories that can be printed. Readers can click on individual words or whole sentences to hear them read aloud as well as record their own voice for later playback of their reading.

- Management tools allow teachers to individualize the program and automatic record keeping is included.

- The software is available in level 1 or level 2.

- The Home Edition is for home use only, and consists of 1 CD that tracks the progress of two learners. Each level costs $210.00

- The School Version is a 2-CD pack. Each CD tracks the progress of 100 learners.

- Windows and Mac

- Each level costs $475.00

English (U.S.) Level 1
by Rosetta Stone, www.rosettastone.com

- The reading comprehension modality of this program can be selected by clicking on the book icon.

- The initial lessons include selecting one of four pictures that match a written word.

- The reading level becomes progressively more difficult.

- The curriculum is carefully sequenced to reinforce existing learning, gradually incorporating new words, phrases, and grammar that is more complex.

- Windows and Mac

- $195.00 for the CD or $49.95 for a one-month online subscription

Fast ForWord
by Scientific Learning Corporation, www.fastforword.com

- Scientific Learning provides a range of products to help with many areas of language.

- It offers programs that feature a sequenced learning environment that advances cognitive skills in the context of appropriate reading skills.

- Providers need to be trained in the use of the software via an online training course that generally takes about five hours.

- $900.00

Lexia Reading Software
by Lexia Learning Systems, www.lexialearning.com

- Lexia offers several programs for different ages that build strength in phonemic awareness, sound-symbol correspondence, decoding, fluency, phonics, and vocabulary.

- Lexia Early Reading is for ages four to six, Lexia Primary Reading is for ages five to eight, and Lexia Strategies is for Older Students Version 4.0 for ages nine to adult.

- The software is based on the Orton-Gillingham method of reading remediation.

- The interactive exercises branch automatically, depending on performance.

- Centralized administration of user data is shared with other Lexia programs and allows teachers and clinicians to track progress. There is complete teacher/clinician control over the selection of program levels, activities, and units for each student.

- Spanish and English directions support ESL learners.

- Windows and Mac

- $159.00 for Strategies for Older Students v4, Family Edition

Merit Software
available from www.meritsoftware.com

- Merit's software products cover the core reading skills.

- Contextual help for users is available at various stages within all Merit programs.

- They integrate text-to-speech technology into reading, grammar, and vocabulary instruction.

- Passages, questions, answers, tips, and explanations can be spoken aloud.

- Windows

- **Reading Comprehension Booster** — Interactive exercises focus on improving the ability to determine the main idea, make inferences, and draw conclusions. Assessments place users in appropriate units of instruction. Immediate instructional feedback is provided. Records can be kept for two users. The home version is $39.00.

- **Developing Critical Thinking Skills for Effective Reading** — Interactive tasks are provided to determine the main idea of a text, select a logical sentence to introduce or complete it, choose an appropriate title to identify it, identify the sequence of details, select an additional supporting sentence, draw an inference, and determine the meaning of unfamiliar words by using other words or phrases in the text as clues. The home version can track performance for two users. $39.00

My House, My Town, and My School: The Language Activities of Daily Living Series
by Laureate Learning Systems, www.laureatelearning.com

- The many levels of this program can be customized for reading practice.

- The program can be set to display the name, description, or function of particular objects.

- The task is for the user to click on the object for which the text is provided.

- It's often helpful for people to work on reading when items are shown in functional scenes.

- Windows and Mac

- $150.00

On Track Reading Series
by Tool Factory, www.toolfactory.com

- Tool Factory's Track Series is a 5 CD set, with each disc isolating a single skill required for the development of fluent reading. Students begin with visual tracking using Eye Track, then work their way forward to formulating complete sentences using Word Track.

- Eye Track provides exercises to develop visual discrimination and spatial orientation, and improve visual figure ground skills. Other activities cover visual discrimination, visual memory, and visual closure.

- Alphabet Track features lessons to help users learn the names of letters, practice alphabetical order, improve short-term memory, and recall alphabetic sequence. Eight self-paced activities are switch-accessible and fully configurable, with selectable colors and multiple levels of difficulty.

- Phoneme Track provides practice with phoneme manipulation, segmentation, and blending.

- Spell Track provides activities for phonemic awareness, left-to-right tracking, word recognition, sequencing, segmenting, blending, and proofreading. Clinicians can add their own word lists and write sentences tailored for each learner.

- Word track shows a sentence on the screen while it is spoken aloud. It then disappears, and the user tracks each word by clicking the correct words, in order, from amongst a string of other words. The appropriate punctuation mark must also be tracked. After tracking, students type the sentence with correct capitalization and punctuation.

- Windows and Mac

- The 5 CDs for a single user cost $299.95. Individual tracks can also be purchased.

Parrot Software Version 8.1
available from www.parrotsoftware.com

- Parrot offers seventy programs with its online subscription for $24.95 per month for Windows. Some of the programs are described below:

  - **Antonym and Synonyms** – A list of words is presented, and the user is first asked to find a word in the list that is the opposite of the target word. Next, the user must find a word in the list that is the same as the target word.

  - **Picture Identification** – A real-life picture is displayed on the screen. A list of three possible names is presented, and the user must select the one that best describes the picture.

  - **Reading Comprehension Adult** – This program targets literal and inferential reading comprehension. Literal items appear verbatim in the story. For errors, the program finds the answer in the story as a strategy for improving comprehension.

  - **Reading Comprehension and Picture Association** – The program presents a short story. After reading the story, the user selects pictures that best answer questions about the story.

  - **Sentence Completion** – An open phrase is displayed at the top of the screen, and the user must select the word that finishes the phrase from three choices listed.

  - **Sorting by Category** – This program requires the user to sort words into related categories.

  - **Traffic Signs** – Clients see one of 112 traffic signs and are presented with three possible descriptions of the sign.

- **Verbal Analogies** — A simple analogy is presented to show a relationship. The first half of an analogy is presented along with five possible choices for completing the analogy.

- **Word Association** — The program presents a word and then asks the client to find an associated word in a list of words.

Reader Rabbit Reading Learning System 2007
by The Learning Company, www.learningcompany.com

- This program was developed for children ages 4-7.

- Activities involve working through puzzles, games, stories and more with Reader Rabbit while practicing reading and language skills.

- There are three interactive adventures:

  - Reader Rabbit road trip

  - Reader Rabbit Wordville Soup

  - Wordville Fair

- Windows and Mac

- $19.99

Reading Detective software
by The Critical Thinking Company, www.criticalthinking.com

- This software develops the analysis, synthesis, and vocabulary skills needed for reading comprehension.

- There are several different versions of this software targeted for different age groups and abilities.

- The activities help users understand reading concepts such as drawing inferences, determining cause and effect, and using context clues to define vocabulary.

- Three levels are provided. Users read and analyze short literature excerpts and stories that include fiction and nonfiction content. They then answer multiple-choice questions, citing sentence-level evidence to support their answers.

- Windows and Mac

- $64.99 for a single-user CD

Simon S.I.O. (Sounds it Out)
by Don Johnson, www.donjohnston.com

- Simon Sounds It Out provides multi-level phonics practice by working on the alphabet, letters, sounds, and words. Users can pick a lesson targeting beginning sounds, ending sounds or both.

- Users learn sounds and build, discriminate, and recall words.

- Animations and graphics reward effort and motivate users to interact with their chosen character.

- There are thirty-one levels of difficulty and built-in single switch scanning is available. Users cannot move to a higher level unless they have completed the previous section to a satisfactory standard.

- Windows and Mac

- $149.00

Thinking Reader
by Tom Snyder Productions, www.tomsnyder.com

- Thinking Reader is a program that systematically builds reading comprehension skills using core, authentic literature.

- It embeds prompts, hints, model answers, and instant feedback into the text to provide individualized instruction.

- Users practice seven scientifically proven reading comprehension strategies while they read.

- Windows and Mac

- $250.00

Time4Learning
by Time4Learning, www.time4learning.com

- Provides home-based online learning from Pre-K to 8th Grade.

- Offers Web-based math and reading programs with interactive curriculum.

- The learn-to-read programs teach and improve phonemic awareness (reading readiness), phonics, reading fluency, vocabulary, and comprehension.

- In upper elementary and middle school, the language arts program teaches reading comprehension, fluency, vocabulary, grammar, pronunciation, punctuation, word roots, literary analysis, and critical thinking.

- Windows and Mac

- $19.95 a month

Understanding Questions Out Loud
by Bungalow Software, www.bungalowsoftware.com

- This program provides practice with understanding various questions: Who? What? When? Where? Why? and How? Auditory cues can be given for support as needed.

- It displays a question and up to four answers. The user reads the question and selects an appropriate response.

- Windows

- $149.50

WordMaker
by Don Johnston, www.donjohnston.com

- This program provides phonics, phonemic-awareness and spelling activities to build core reading strategies.

- Students manipulate letters to make words to help discover their patterns, and then sort the words into rhymes and use the rhymes to decode and spell new words. 140 lessons give users word manipulation practice. Windows and Mac

- $149.00

Refer to Chapters 16 and 17 in this guide for additional suggestions regarding the use of multimedia software and many online resources with games, exercises, pictures, and adapted newspapers to improve reading comprehension.

Software for Vision-Based Reading Deficits

According to the National Center for Learning Disabilities (www.ncld.org), a visual processing, or perceptual, disorder refers to a hindered ability to make sense of information taken in through the eyes. This is different from problems involving sight or sharpness of vision. Difficulties with visual processing affect how visual information is interpreted or processed by the brain. People with visual deficits often

- reverse and invert letters,

- avoid reading,

- have difficulty copying written material,

- reread and skip lines,

- lose their space while reading,

- complain that print blurs while reading,

- turn their head while reading,

- hold their paper at odd angles to read,

- close one eye to read,

- have difficulty recognizing an object or word if only part of it is shown,

- misalign letters, and/or

- have messy papers.

Clients who have visual-perceptual deficits or low vision can often benefit from the use of text-to-speech or screen-reading software, which is described in the next section. Many programs highlight words and sentences as they are read aloud and work to help improve visual-perceptual skills. The highlighting can help with scanning and tracking the written words. In addition to the software described below, several non-tech strategies can help improve reading. Low-tech strategies to help with visual-based deficits include using large-print books or a magnifying glass, and providing tracking tools such as a ruler and lines. Make sure that clients are wearing reading glasses if they have them, and provide a workspace that is free of clutter.

Title	Web Site	Price	PC	Mac	Other
EyeQ	www.infmind.com	CD $199.00 Per month online $49.95	x	x	Online
Eye Track	www.toolfactory.com	$69.95	x	x	
High Level Attention	www.learningfundamentals.com	$99.99	x	x	
Lexia Cross-Trainer Visual-Spatial	www.lexialearning.com	$298.00	x	x	
RedBar	www.bungalowsoftware.com	$119.50	x		
Smart Driver	www.braintrain.com	$258.00	x		

EyeQ
by Infinite Mind, www.infmind.com

- This is a high-level speed-reading program that is helpful for clients who have subtle visual-perceptual deficits.

- There are twelve seven-minute sessions designed to strengthen the users' eyes, widen their field of vision, and increase reading speed.

- The EyeQ program may help improve comprehension. When readers read faster, they have time to use the preview-read-review method described in the program. This improves comprehension and makes reading more efficient.

- Users are able to adjust the column width, font size, and reading speed to match reading preferences.

- The Web edition is available for several different lengths of time. Thirty days is $49.95.

- Windows and Mac

- $199.95 for the CD version

Eye Track
by Tool Factory, www.toolfactory.com

- Eye Track is designed to train visual perception skills. Visual information is presented in a variety of ways to work on visual recognition, recall, discrimination, and meaning of visual input.

- This software is most appropriate for children.

- Windows or Mac

- $69.95

High Level Attention
by Learning Fundamentals, www.learningfundamentals.com

- This module is part of the Attention and Memory: Volume I CD and is available as a separate CD.

- One game on the CD is called "Catch of the Day." Its goal is to improve visual scanning and identification as the complexity of the visual field increases.

- The user clicks on numbers embedded in a field of alphabet letters.

- This program may be used to train compensatory strategies for hemianopsia and left-side neglect.

- There are thirteen levels of difficulty.

- Windows and Mac

- $99.00

Lexia Cross-Trainer Visual-Spatial
by Lexia Learning, www.lexialearning.com

- Lexia Cross-Trainer: Visual-Spatial works on different kinds of "muscles": visualization, visual memory, mental rotation, visual tracking, spatial orientation, and multi-perspective coordination, among other skills.

- Windows and Mac

- The family edition is $298.00.

RedBar
by Bungalow Software, www.bungalowsoftware.com

- RedBar software helps clients who have left or right neglect.

- At designated intervals, it trains users to notice (or "attend to") their left or right side. If they don't click on the arrow that appears on the side of the screen that the client often ignores, RedBar gives them a stronger reminder.

- If they still fail to click the side, it shows a black arrow from in their intact visual field to guide them to the challenging side of the screen. The software works best when used in conjunction with another program, such as a word processor or while reading e-mail.

- Windows

- $119.50

SmartDriver
by Brain Train at www.braintrain.com

- SmartDriver is a non-violent, driving game designed to improve visual tracking skills, hand-eye coordination, planning, attention to detail, concentration, memory, and patience.

- To win the game, the user needs to drive a car successfully through progressively more difficult roads and driving situations.

- Windows

- SmartDriver packaged with Steering Wheel with Brake & Accelerator Pedals is $258.00

Computer Accommodations for People With Visual-Perceptual Deficits

There are many options available for people with visual impairments that come already available on many computers. Many of these computer adaptations have been discussed in Chapters 5 and 6 of this guide.

Personal Computers

Computers that use a Windows operating system come with many accessibility options built-in. Users with low vision often depend on the ability to enlarge or enhance on-screen information. More detailed information can be found at www.microsoft.com/enable. To make on-screen information easier to see and to understand, use the display screens under the control panel on Windows-based computers.

- Change the font style, color, and size of items on the desktop — Using the display options, choose font color, size, and style combinations.

- Change the icon size — Make icons larger for visibility or smaller for increased screen space.

- Alter screen resolution — Change pixel count to enlarge objects on screen.

- Provide high-contrast schemes — Select color combinations that are easier to see.

- Adjust cursor width and blink rate — Make the cursor easier to locate, or eliminate the distraction of its blinking.

- Use a Microsoft Magnifier — Enlarge portion of screen for better visibility.

- Use text-to-speech — Narrator is a basic text-to-speech utility that reads what is displayed on the screen, i.e., the contents of the active window, menu options, or text that has been typed.

Macintosh Computers

There are options built-into Macintosh computers. Detailed information can be found at www.apple.com/education/accessibility/disabilities/vision.

Solutions for people with visual impairments include the following options:

- Zoom — this feature includes a number of options, like the ability to set maximum and minimum values for rapid zooming in and out, a preview rectangle that outlines the portion of the screen that will be magnified, and the ability to customize how the screen moves as you navigate with the mouse pointer.

- Change cursor size — Mac OS X enables you to easily increase the size of the mouse cursor, so it's easier to find and follow when you move the mouse.

- Text-to-speech — VoiceOver is a fully integrated, built-in screen reader technology providing access to the Mac through speech, audible cues, and keyboard navigation. Text-to-Speech Synthesis allows users to hear text read aloud. Simply select Speech from the Services menu of most applications, and hear the computer start speaking.

- Visual display — View Options enables the user to increase icon size and text size for icons. Flexible display adjustments provide users with visually appealing options, such as a white-on-black display.

There are also quite a few programs on the market to assist people with low vision. It's beyond the scope of this guide to review them all.

Additional information can be found on the following Web sites:

- www.lowvision.org
- www.enablemart.com
- www.independentliving.com

Assistive Reading Technology

Assistive reading technologies may help with the following:

- Improving skills related to decoding, reading fluency, and comprehension by reading the text aloud.

- Transferring written material that is not in digital format into the computer using Optical Character Recognition (OCR), so that the text-to-speech software can read it aloud.

- Using alternative book formats such as "e-books" and "talking books."

- Improving strategies for synthesizing written information with the help of reading guides.

- Supporting reading, studying, writing, and electronic file management through the use of advanced talking word-processing software which is discussed in Chapter 13, "Treatment and Technology To Improve Written Expression."

Many assistive technology tools are available to help people who struggle with reading. For a review of some of the technologies, refer to the following Web site: www.ebookmall.com/aboutebooks.htm.

Optical Character Recognition (OCR) and Text-to-Speech

Software with text-to-speech capabilities can read aloud text on a computer screen. This multi-sensory input is very helpful for reading. It's visually engaging and increases reading speed, comprehension, and retention.

There are quite a few text-to-speech products on the market. This software may include the following features:

- The ability to control auditory features and visual presentation.
- The ability to save the documents as auditory files that can be downloaded to handheld devices.
- Options, such as voice, rate of speech, highlighting, and screen display, may be individualized, depending on the software.
- Text that can be read back a letter, word, line, sentence, or paragraph at a time.
- Words that can be magnified as they are read aloud.
- The ability to work with e-mail, Web sites, and Microsoft Word and PDF documents.

Basic Programs

Universal Reader by Premiere Assistive Technology, NextUp! by NextUp.com, Read Please 2003 by Read Please, and WordQ2 by Quillsoft are a few of the relatively inexpensive, easy-to-use text-reading software programs for e-mailing and basic word processing.

Full-Featured Programs With Text to Speech

There are times when individuals with more complex reading needs would benefit from an advanced talking word processor with study and writing support. These might include Kurzweil 3000 by Kurzweil Educational Systems, Read and Write Gold by TextHelp, Wynn Wizard by Freedom Scientific, and the Talking Word Processor by Premiere Assistive Technology. These programs provide helpful support for clients who will be typing extensively and who need help with organization and studying.

Users can

- electronically highlight sections of text in different colors,
- take notes by typing or by voice,

- prepare outlines,
- create flashcards and other study materials,
- read only highlighted sections, and
- skip to the bookmarked section of text.

Optical Character Recognition

Optical Character Recognition (OCR) enables a user to scan printed material into a computer or handheld unit. The software converts the "image" to text, so a text-reading program can read the written material to the user. Different programs use different scan and OCR engines. Certain programs work best with certain scanners. Also, some work better than others with replication of the image, scanning speed, form-filling capabilities, and study skills.

Assistive Technology Software Programs for Reading Support

Title	Web Site	Price	PC	Mac	Other
2nd Speech Center v3.00	www.2ndspeechcenter.com	$39.95	x		
ClipRead	www.clipread.com	Per year $34.95	x		Online subscription
E-Text Reader 3.0	www.readingmadeeasy.com	$39.95	x		
FSReader	www.freedomscientific.com	$79.95	x		
Key to Access	www.readingmadeeasy.com	$399.95	x		
KNFB Reader	www.knfreader.com www.envisiontechnoology.com	$3,495.00			Hand-held device
Kurzweil 3000 for Windows Version 11	www.kurzweiledu.com	$1,495.00	x	x	
LiveInk	www.liveink.com				For research
Microsoft Narrator	www.microsoft.com	Free with Windows	x		

Title	Web Site	Price	PC	Mac	Other
Microsoft Text-to-Speech Package	www.microsoft.com	Free download	x		
Mobile Speak Pocket	www.codefactory.com	$499.00			Pocket PC
Pocket Hal	www.yourdolphin.com	$595.00			Pocket PC
Pocket Reader	www.ablelinktech.com	$199.00			Pocket PC
Read:OutLoud Solo Edition	www.donjohnston.com	$299.00	x	x	
ReadPlease 2003	www.readplease.com	Free download	x		
ReadPlease Plus 2003	www.readplease.com	$59.95	x		
Reading Pens	www.wizcomtech.com	$279.00			Hand-held Device
ReadingBar 2 for Internet Explorer	www.readplease.com	$79.95	x		
TextAloud	www.nextup.com	$29.95	x		
UltraHall Text to Speech Screen Reader	www.zabaware.com	$24.95	x		
Universal Reader 4.0	www.readingmadeeasy.com	$39.95	x		
VisioVoice 1.0.1	www.assistiveware.com	$185.00		x	
VoiceOver	www.apple.com	Free with Macs		x	
WordQ 2	www.clipread.com	$185.00	x		

2nd Speech Center v3.00
by 2nd Speech Center, www.2ndspeechcenter.com

- This software enables the user to listen to documents, e-mails, or Web pages.
- It also allows for the conversion of text to MP3 or WAV files for listening later on an MP3 player.
- It supports dozens of voices including AT&T Natural Voices, for over eleven languages.
- Windows
- $39.95

ClipRead
by Walker Reading Technologies, www.clipread.com

- ClipRead is a software application that enables readers to submit text via the Internet to powerful engines that reformat the text in a way that makes it easier to read and easier to understand,
- It converts most a digital text to LiveInk which takes out the graphics. (Refer to description of LivInk below.)
- Windows
- The subscription price is $34.95 a year.

E-Text Reader 3.0
by Premiere Assistive Technology, www.readingmadeeasy.com

- This reader offers the ability to change voices, to read at any speed, and to make notes into the document you're reading. The reader can highlight with four different colors.
- Users are able to extract all text highlighted in a color and save to separate files for review.
- The format of the extracted information is retained during the extraction, including graphics that are part of the highlighted text.
- Windows
- 39.95

FSReader
by Freedom Scientific, www.freedomscientific.com

- Allows users to access audio material available from Recording for the Blind & Dyslexic (RFB&D).

- Users can read and navigate digital talking books and e-books produced in the Digital Accessible Information System (DAISY) format on a desktop or laptop PC.

- Features are offered to view a book by browsing headings or flipping pages, setting multiple bookmarks, and resuming reading where a book was left off when the program was closed. In books that contain audio narration, users can fast forward, rewind, and adjust the speed of the narrator.

- To access RFB&D's AudioPlus books with FSReader, users need a special User Authorization Key (UAK) obtained by calling 800-221-4792.

- Windows

- $79.95

Key to Access
by Premiere Assistive Technology, www.readingmadeeasy.com

- Key to Access enables a client's assistive reading tools to be used on any computer without loading the software onto the computer. The software is installed on a portable USB MP3 player.

- By just inserting the MP3 player into any USB port, the floating toolbar will appear and then you select any of the eight different tools. Personal settings are saved on your Key to Access.

- The built-in voice recorder allows the user to dictate notes or record lectures and listen to them later.

- It include the following programs:

  - **Scan and Read Pro** — scanning software that allows you to capture hard-copy materials in a digital format and then reads them to you

  - **Universal Reader Plus** — helpful for reading and writing e-mails and reading Web pages

  - **E-Text Reader** — a study tool that allows you to highlight, bookmark, search, and extract text from a document

  - **Ultimate Talking Dictionary** — a 250,000-word dictionary with integrated thesaurus

  - **Talking Word Processor** — a talking word processor, talking word prediction, and a talking grammar check

- **PDF Magic** — software that can convert inaccessible PDF files to accessible formats

- **Text to Audio** — Assists with the conversion of digital documents to MP3 format and puts them right on your Key to Access player, so that they can be listened to away from the computer

- **Onscreen Talking Calculator**

- Windows

- $399.95

KNFB Reader
by KNFB Reading Technology, www.knfreader.com (also available at www.envisiontechnology.org)

- This is a new handheld device that combines a digital camera with a personal data assistant (PDA) housed in a custom-designed case.

- Uses character recognition with text-to-speech technology in a mobile solution that will magnify text and read it aloud.

- The user holds the Reader over print — a restaurant menu, a memo for work, print material on the wall — and takes a picture. In seconds, the content of the printed document is read aloud in clear synthetic speech.

- The information can be read and discarded, or stored to read later or transferred to a computer.

- $3,495.00

Kurzweil 3000 for Windows Version 11
by Kurzweil Educational Systems, www.kurzweiledu.com (also available at www.envisiontechnology.org)

- This program reads aloud electronic or scanned text and provides support for writing and studying with active learning, studying, and test-taking strategies.

- It simultaneously highlights and reads aloud the text with a variable rate of speech, providing the user with customizable visual tracking and auditory presentation. These features are especially helpful for people with low vision and slow auditory processing.

- The user can click on a word in the body of the text to get a definition or synonym or decode the word into syllables and spell out the letters.

- It is fluent in Spanish, French, German, Italian, and Dutch.

- Kurzweil offers both a license-to-go and remote license-to-go, so that users can access the program while using a computer that is not connected to a Kurzweil 3000 Network. This option is useful for clients using Kurzweil 3000 on a home computer that cannot be brought to school.

- The Kurzweil 3000 taskbar gives students access to Kurzweil 3000 reading, word lookup, and spell-check tools when working in other applications such as Microsoft Word.

- The broadcast feature lets the user use the Server Administrator software to disable, enable, or leave "as is" selected Kurzweil 3000 features on multiple client computers. This makes it helpful to administer tests, protect documents, or provide consistency for user interfaces.

- An appointment calendar in included with audible reminders.

- Kurzweil can send files to handheld devices, so you can read and reference important material when away from your home or office computer.

- It includes a classic literature CD containing hundreds of titles of electronic text.

- Windows and Mac

- A single professional color version is $1,495.00.

LiveInk
by Open Text Products, www liveink.com

- LiveInk provides the user with text-to-speech; and the ability to change font size, font color, spacing, and background color all make digital text a powerful tool for people with print disabilities.

- It is based on scientific discoveries in syntax and vision. LiveInk arranges text into meaningful, visually friendly phrase patterns.

- Live Ink's text-analysis and enhanced display methods, and associated software, are globally-patented intellectual property that is available for licensing by publishers, technology companies, and educational, governmental, and commercial institutions that produce and use electronic text.

- It is only available for research and software use.

- For more information contact rwalker@liveink.com.

Microsoft Narrator
by Microsoft Corporation, www.microsoft.com

- Narrator is a light-duty screen reader utility that is included with Microsoft Windows 2000 and Windows XP computers.

- It reads dialog boxes and window controls in a number of the more basic applications for Windows.

- It is not intended to be a fully functioning screen reader. Narrator can assist a blind person in installing a full-function screen reader, assisting the user until his or her screen reader of choice is up and running.

- Free with Windows

Microsoft Text-to-Speech Package
by Microsoft Corporation, www.microsoft.com

- This program can be downloaded for free from www.microsoft.com.

- Microsoft Reader is available for tablet PCs, Windows-based PCs, and laptops.

- This software enables computer users to access e-books.

Mobile Speak Pocket
by Code Factory, www.codefactory.com

- Mobile Speak Pocket is screen-reading software for pocket PC devices.

- Complete access to the applications on a pocket PC device such as Internet Explorer, Messaging, MSN Messenger, Calendar, Contacts, Tasks, Notes, Pocket Word, Pocket Excel, and Windows Media Player is available.

- $499.00 at www.enablemart.com

Pocket Hal
by Dolphin at www.yourdolphin.com – available in the US at Freedom of Speech, Assistive Technology Solutions, http://fos.stores.yahoo.net

- Pocket Hal is a new Pocket PC screen reader that was developed for the Windows Mobile operating system that is available on PDAs and PDA phones.

- $595.00

Pocket Reader
by AbleLink Technologies, www.ablelinktech.com

- Pocket Reader enables non-readers to access previously inaccessible reading materials or education and recreation.

- It uses a mainstream Pocket PC platform to encourage inclusion.

- Books can be accessed from www.audible.com.

- There is a low vision mode.

- $199.00

Read:OutLoud Solo Edition
by Don Johnston Incorporated, www.donjohnston.com

- Read:OutLoud is a text reader that supports individuals with modeling, scaffolding, and practice of reading strategies to comprehend text. It is geared toward the school-age population.

- It is helpful to also purchase Start-to-Finish Core Content, which is also provided by Don Johnston, for $79.00

- This software can also be purchased in a bundle with other software that assists with writing, such as Don Johnston's Draft:Builder and Co:Writer.

- Windows and Mac

- The cost is $299.00

ReadPlease 2003
by Read Please, www.readplease.com

- This free download uses Microsoft voices, reads text from any program via Windows Clipboard, offers an adjustable voice speed, and can customize font and background color.

- The interface is easy to use, with VCR-like controls.

ReadPlease Plus 2003
by Read Please, www.readplease.com

- In addition to the features of ReadPlease 2003, this product allows the user to add words and pronunciations; start playback anywhere in a document; use a low-vision or large-controls option; navigate forward and backward in the document; highlight text while reading; and use a dock mode to keep the toolbar at the top of the screen.

- There is an adjustable pause between paragraphs and hot-key controls for all functions.

- It's compatible with AT&T Natural Voices, and more languages are available.

- Windows

- $59.95

Reading Pens
by Wizcom Technologies at www.wizcomtech.com

- There are several portable scanners and pens that use text-to-speech software to offer word by word pronunciation of scanned words, lines of text, definitions and synonyms through an integrated speaker or headphones.

- They generally require good manual dexterity, vision, and cognitive skills for functional use.

- Pens differ in their scanning speeds. Prices vary depending on selected features.

- The Basic Reading Pen costs $279.00

ReadingBar 2 for Internet Explorer
by Read Please, www.readplease.com

- ReadingBar 2 reads any Web page aloud, highlights words in Internet Explorer, creates MP3 or WAV files from Web pages, generates a text-only version from any Web page, and can use a reader window.

- It also magnifies pages, text, pictures, and scrollbars, translates Web pages into four languages, and offers use of a dictionary.

- The user can edit the pronunciation of words.

- It uses Microsoft Voices and is compatible with AT&T Voices.

- $79.95

TextAloud by NextUp
available from www.nextup.com

- This software reads text aloud from e-mail, Web pages, and written documents.

- TextAloud can also save the audio file to MP3 or Windows Media files ready for playback on an iPod, a Pocket PC, or a TV with Tivo's Home Media Option.

- It uses the AT&T and NeoSpeech voices. In the summer of 2006, it partnered with Acapela Group to bring twenty new 22 kHz voices, available in ten languages.

- There is a multi-article mode that uses a dropdown list showing titles of all articles and allowing article switching at the top of the window.

- Toolbar options allow the user to change the size of the toolbar icons and choose whether the toolbar will have captions or not. The user can also change the look and color scheme of the TextAloud window.

- A visible speed-control slider allows the user to make adjustments to the currently selected voice, even while speaking is underway.

- A hot key can be used for proofreading.

- Windows

- $29.95

UltraHal Text to Speech Screen Reader with Neo Speech Voice Text
by Zabaware, www.zabaware.com

- The Ultra Hal Text-to-Speech Reader application will read your documents aloud in one of its many high quality voices.

- This program can be used for proof reading, reading e-book, standard Windows dialog box message, and clipboard contents. With this function, you can easily have it read your e-mail and Web sites.

- This program is also able to speak incoming instant messages aloud and convert text files into WAVE audio files.

- Windows

- $24.95

Universal Reader 4.0
by Premiere Assistive Technology, www.readingmadeeasy.com

- Universal Reader software reads aloud selected text to the user.

- It can be used to read e-mail, Word documents, and Web pages.

- The user clicks on the "mouth" icon to read, the "stoplight" to stop, the "yellow light" to pause, and the "rewind button" to start over from the beginning.

- The program highlights the word as it is read.

- To make viewing easier, the text can be changed and enlarged, and colors can be altered.

- With the "talking pointer," the user can place the cursor over virtually any online text, icon, or picture and the text or a description of the image will be read aloud without clicking, cutting and pasting, or highlighting.

- There is a choice of voices and speeds.

- A "Plus" version comes with scanning capabilities.

- Windows

- $39.95

VisioVoice 1.0.1
by AssistiveWare at www.assistiveware.com

- VisioVoice 1.0.1 is a newly released product for Mac users providing a number of speech and vision related features to enhance access to Mac OS X.

- It can convert Text, Word, HTML, PDF and RTF files to audio files or iPod-ready iTunes tracks.

- There are large cross hairs and cursors, and a text and image zoom window.

- Words are spoken aloud as they are highlighted.
- There is multilingual support.
- Mac
- $185.00

VoiceOver
by Apple Computers at www.apple.com

- VoiceOver is a screen reader that is included on the Mac OS X computer.
- This accessibility interface offers magnification options, keyboard control, and spoken English descriptions of what's happening on screen.
- VoiceOver reads aloud the contents of files, including Web pages, mail messages, and word processing files, and provides a comprehensive audible description of the workspace, such as keyboard commands for interacting with application and system controls.
- Press Command-F5 to activate VoiceOver and then audible prompts instruct the user how to use it.
- Included with Mac OS X computers.

WordQ 2
by Quillsoft, www.wordq.com

- WordQ is a software tool used along with standard writing software.
- It reads selected text aloud and has a word prediction component that can be used with writing.
- It can read aloud letters, words, and sentences—or an entire document.
- A variety of voices are available, and the speed at which the text is read can be controlled.
- This software can be used with SpeakQ, which is a simplified word recognition software discussed in Chapter 11, "Treatment and Technology To Improve Written Expression."
- Windows
- $185.00

Alternative Reading Formats

Resources for Recorded Books

Recorded books allow users to listen to text. They are available in a variety of formats, such as audiocassettes, CDs, and MP3 downloads. Subscription services offer extensive electronic library collections.

Recording for the Blind and Dyslexic (RFB&D)
available at **www.rfbd.org**

- This is a nonprofit service organization that provides educational books (academic textbooks) on audiocassette and CD.

- It also offers a large collection of nonfiction books.

- The service for schools requires a $50.00 registration fee and a $25.00 membership service charge a year. Individual memberships are $65.00 for the initial fee and $35.00 a year.

National Library Service for the Blind and Physically Handicapped (NLS)
available at www.loc.gov/nls

- This is a free service of the Library of Congress that is commonly referred to as "Talking Books."

- NLS offers leisure materials and magazines on an audiocassette or audio disk. The collection includes popular novels, classical literature, poetry, biographies, and magazines.

- Talking Books are distributed through a network of regional and sub-regional libraries.

Resources for E-Text

An increasing number of books are available in e-text format. The book's content may be available on a CD, by scanning with optical character recognition (OCR) or by Internet download. One benefit of this format is the ability to change the appearance of the text. The way the reader sees the text can have a profound impact on comprehension. Cluttered pages, with little white space and small print, make reading more difficult. With e-text, it's often helpful to enlarge the font and increase the color contrast of the text and background to make on-screen reading easier. When text is provided electronically, it can be imported into text readers and talking word processors.

The Accessible Book Collection
available at www.accessiblebookcollection.org

- This is a subscription-based service with over 500 books with a high-interest, low reading level. It offers detailed information on the reading level for each title. The primary audience is youth with learning disabilities. Intellipics and Clicker formatted picture books are now available. They offer tools so that the text size, color, and spacing of their e-books can be changed. District site licenses are available. Individuals are eligible if they have a documented disability that prevents them from reading standard print effectively. The cost of an annual subscription is $49.95.

Bookshare.org
available at www.bookshare.org

- This subscription-based online service provides thousands of digital books to people with disabilities. It also includes many newspapers and magazines. This service provides more access to recreational reading material than RFB&D. Any subscriber can obtain public domain books in text and HTML format, with which they can use their own text-to-speech software. The setup fee is $25.00; the annual fee of $50.00 allows members to download as many books as desired.

Project Gutenberg
available at www.gutenberg.org

- Project Gutenberg is the first and largest single collection of free electronic books. Its founder, Michael Hart, invented e-books in 1971. The project offers seventeen thousand free books, which were produced by hundreds of volunteers.

Digital Book Index
available at www.digitalbookindex.org

- The Digital Book Index provides links to more than 114,000 title records from more than 1,800 commercial and noncommercial publishers, universities, and various private sites. About 75,000 of the books, texts, and documents are available free, and many others are available at a modest cost.

E-Book Mall
available at www-ebookmall.com

- Includes over 150,000 e-books for purchase.

NewsLink
available at www.newslink.org

- This site includes links to more than 4,000 U.S. online newspapers, magazines, and news and talk radio stations.

Onlinenewspapers.com
available at www.onlinenewspapers.com

- This site links to thousands of world newspapers for free.

Interactive Talking Books

Many mainstream and specialized interactive talking books can improve reading skills. They may be software to use on the computer, or combined with other technology devices. In addition to these products, please refer to Chapter 16, "Multi-Media Programs and Generating Printed Treatment Materials," to learn to create Talking Books for your clients.

Living Books Software
by The Learning Company, available at www.learningcompany.com

- Young readers listen to the text and play games to improve word pronunciation, reading comprehension, vocabulary and computer literacy.

- Many titles are available, such as *Arthur* and *Stellaluna*.

- Switch users can turn pages by clicking on the switch when the pointer is placed on the arrow which moves the book to the next page.

- Living Books Library School Edition is includes seven stories for $250.00.

LeapPad and Leapster Electronic Books
by LeapPad Learning System at www.leapfrog.com

- Special books and cartridges are used with a player.

- A special pen is used to interact with the book with a variety of activities to improve reading and cognition. Sounds, words, sentences and definitions can be said aloud by the player.

- There are over 50 titles for different ages.

- The starter pack for the Leapster Learning System is $59.99. Additional cartridge/games are approximately $24.99.

- The starter pack for the LeapPad Plus Writing Learning System is $39.97.

Adapted Online Newspapers

News-2-You
available at www.news-2-you.com

- This is an Internet-based picture newspaper that features current events and other articles of interest.

- There are three editions: regular, simplified, and higher.

- Communication boards can also be downloaded each week.

- Written exercises are provided for reading comprehension practice.

- Typically, crossword puzzles, matching activities, and multiple-choice questions are also provided.

- This newspaper is an ideal source for material for communication groups and as a resource for family members who are looking for fresh and relevant therapy content.

- The cost is $79.00 for a single subscription for one year.

NewsCurrents
Available at www.newscurrents.com

- NewsCurrents is a current events newspaper with accompanying discussion guides.

- It's written on three levels of difficulty and is available online or on DVD.

- A subscription includes a weekly issue (for thirty-four weeks of the year) with images corresponding to five or six stories in that week's news.

- There is a mailed printed teacher's guide that contains topic discussion suggestions and visuals to generate helpful current events sessions, as well as Web sites for additional research.

- A senior version for adults is available.

- The price varies from $99.00 to $309.00

Special English from Voice of America
Available at www.voanews.com/specialenglish

- Special English From Voice of America is an online newspaper. Clients can listen to the story read aloud, and watch a person speaking at the same time as reading the text.

- Material is provided which reports world events and describing discoveries in medicine and science.

- This online newspaper is written in short, simple sentences that contain only one idea. No idioms are used. It has a limited vocabulary of 1,500 words. Most are simple words that describe objects, actions, or emotions, although some are more difficult.

- The material is spoken at a slower pace, about two-thirds the speed of Standard English for increased comprehension.

- Special English broadcasts around the world seven days a week, five times a day. Each half-hour broadcast begins with ten minutes of the latest news followed by twenty minutes of feature programming.

- There is a different short feature every weekday about science, development, agriculture, and environment, and on the weekend, about news events and American idioms.

- Free

BookBox
available at www.bookbox.com

- This resource is most appropriate for children.

- There are downloadable Flash stories that are digitally narrated with simple animation and streaming text across the bottom.

- It synchronizes the text, audio, and visual media to create an educational and entertaining reading experience.

- The reader sees whole phrases, and the letters go from white to red as the words are spoken.

- The stories are available in multiple languages.

- Many stories are available for download for $1.99 each. CDs with several stories are approximately $12.99.

Reading Pens and Portable Spell Checkers

Reading pens and portable spell checkers can be used when a reader can decode most text, but needs help with limited words.

Reading Pen 11
available at www.wizcom.com or resellers such as www.enablemart.com, www.quick-pen.com, and www.accessingenuity.com

- There are quite a few different types of reading pens available.

- Individual words are enlarged on the display, and words may be spelled out, or broken into syllables. This Pen is a completely portable self-contained device and does not require a computer.

- It assists users by providing a definition of the scanned word or line of text, as well as reading both the words and definition aloud using text-to-speech technology.

- The Reading Pen contains over 480,000 words from the American Heritage® College Dictionary, 3rd Edition.

- For some users it is challenging to hold it steady and move it smoothly across a page.

- A "training foot" can be purchased for added stability.

- It sometimes helps to start at the end and scan backwards.

- $279.95

Speaking Homework Wiz
available at www.franklin.com, and at stores such as www.bestbuy.com and
www.staples.com

- This Franklin product speaks letters, words, and definitions.

- Users can program personal word lists.

- When users have difficulty reading a word, they can type it into this device
  and hear it aloud.

- Word games are included.

- $59.95

Low-Tech Visual Aides

- **Color** — Written items can be color-coded with a with highlighter or
  removable highlighting tape, so they are easy to find visually. Using a system
  of different colors for different types of information can help cue users to
  where to look for text.

- **Marking Presentation Material** — Specific markers can also be used to
  indicate new sections, places to start, directions, or important information to
  remember. Sticky notes, page flags, and reading guides are also helpful and
  do not lift print or otherwise damage

Chapter 13:
Treatment and Technology To Improve Written Expression

People who have had strokes and head injuries, degenerative diseases, language/learning disabilities and other communication, cognitive and physical challenges often have difficulty with one or more aspects of written language. There may be issues related to the following tasks:

- Maintaining attention to the task
- Retrieving words
- Sequencing the words into sentences
- Using proper grammar and syntax
- Spelling correctly
- Organizing the written content
- Initiating writing activities
- Physically writing with a pencil or pen and typing

Before considering technology options, a variety of positioning alternatives and low-tech options should be tried. Examples of low-tech options include: slant boards, alternative pens and pencils, pencil grips, and special writing paper. If these strategies are not successful, it may then be time to consider assistive technology to help with written expression and the physical act of putting words onto the paper.

A few online sources for these low-tech options for improving written expression are the following companies:

- Onion Mountain Technology, Inc., www.onionmountaintech.com
- Therapro, Inc., www.theraproducts.com

Computer-based solutions do not work for all individuals. Many find the computer environment confusing, complex, and frustrating. As with other therapy goals, most new users will require initial training and support for using the software, and in some cases continuing support may be needed.

People with written language challenges may have difficulty with one or more aspects of written language. These trouble spots might include

- the proper use of grammar and syntax,

- punctuation,

- spelling, and/or

- organizational skills.

This chapter will discuss the following strategies and resources for improved writing:

- Software with customizable drill-and-practice exercises to improve writing

- Software to improve spelling

- Software to help stimulate written content

- Features of word processors and assistive writing technology

- Text-based word processing features

- Text- based word processors

- Picture-based talking word processors

- Stand-alone word prediction and word bank programs

- Dictionaries

- Graphic organizers: technology for organizing written narrative

- Technology to help with the physical aspect of writing

- Speech-to-text and voice recognition

- Initiation of the writing process

- The physical act of handwriting or typing

- Portable word processors

Software With Customizable Drill-and-Practice Exercises To Improve Writing

There is quite a bit of software patterned in a drill-and-practice format. Such programs don't replace worksheets and workbook tasks, which still have value because typing and writing by hand are both valuable skills. However, the benefits of software use are many, as discussed in Chapter 1, "Why Use Technology?"

- Software for children typically stimulates them to practice a variety of skills disguised through graphic games and activities.

- Products for adults are typically more straightforward. These applications reinforce the need for repeated skills practice for people with writing difficulty.

- Quite a few programs are aimed at improving copying words and sentences, written confrontation naming, and phrase- and sentence-level written expression.

- There are programs targeted toward improving grammar, spelling, and punctuation.

- Many products on the market teach keyboarding skills, but they are not the focus of this guide.

Clinicians need to customize the tasks for each individual. Programs differ in the techniques and reinforcements they use toward establishing improved writing skills. Characteristics for software selection were discussed in Chapter 5.

- Programs vary in the options that are available for individualized practice.

- The same program with the same options may be used in different ways with different clients to maximize the quality of that person's practice toward established goals.

- Correct responses are rewarded with a positive comment or graphic display.

- Incorrect responses are typically followed by guidance toward selecting the correct answer.

- If several incorrect responses are given by the client, it's best if the program provides assistance toward eliciting the correct response or provides a way for the client to view the correct answer.

- Programs that do not provide help toward the correct response are often frustrating for clients when they get "stuck." However, they may become more appropriate as the client improves.

- Additional features of some drill-and-practice programs include a performance record, a main menu from which to select a variety of lessons, multiple-choice drills, and typing lessons in which the user is asked to type a correct word, letter, or sentence.

Title	Web Site	Price	PC	Mac	Other
Aphasia Tutor 1+: Words Out Loud	www.bungalowsoftware.com	$199.00	x		
Aphasia Tutor 2+: Sentences Out Loud	www.bungalowsoftware.com	$199.00	x		
Editor in Chief - Beginning	www.criticalthinking.com	$64.99	x	x	

Title	Web Site	Price	PC	Mac	Other
English U.S. Level 1	www.rosettastone.com	$195.00 Per month online $49.95	x	x	Online subscription
Grammar Fitness	www.meritsoftware.com	$129.00	x		
My House and My Town	www.laureatelearning.com	$150.00	x	x	
No-Glamour Grammar	www.lingusystems.com	$41.95	x	x	
Paragraph Punch	www.meritsoftware.com	$149.99	x		
Parrot Software	www.parrotsoftware.com	Per month online $24.94	x		Online subscription
Punctuation Puzzler	www.criticalthinking.com	$59.99	x	x	
WriteAssist	www.secondguessusa.com	$119.00	x		
C-Pen 20	www.cpenusa.com	$149.00			Hand-held scanner

Aphasia Tutor 1+: Words Out Loud and Aphasia Tutor 2+: Sentences Out Loud
by Bungalow Software, www.bungalowsoftware.com

- Aphasia Tutor 1+: Words Out Loud and Aphasia Tutor 2+: Sentences Out Loud are customizable programs with many lessons of varying levels to improve written word retrieval skills and writing ability at the word and sentence levels.

- To improve writing, there are letter, word, phrase, sentence, and definition completion fill-ins.

- As the client is typing a response, the computer provides visual feedback regarding correct and incorrect letters written.

- There is a "Show Hint" button that indicates the number of letters in the target response.

- If the client is unable to type the word, the entire text is displayed, and it becomes a copying task.

- Auditory as well as visual cues may be provided as needed.

- Windows

- $199.00 for each professional version

Editor in Chief -Beginning
by Critical Thinking Co., www.criticalthinking.com

- Editor in Chief is a program to help improve grammar, punctuation, spelling, capitalization, and attention to detail using a standards-based thinking approach.

- This method teaches the writer to analyze and edit stories that contain errors in writing mechanics and story details.

- There are many different levels available for purchase.

- Users identify and click on errors in each story and then select the category and specific rule that applies to each error.

- Windows and Mac

- $64.99

English U.S. Level 1
by Rosetta Stone, www.rosettastone.com

- This program offers written expression lessons when the keyboard icon is selected. The program progresses in syntactic difficulty, and lessons are grouped by functional topic.

- The user writes what is heard, and the computer provides feedback pertaining to the spelling, syntax, and punctuation.

- The curriculum is sequenced, gradually incorporating new words, phrases, and more complex grammar as it reinforces existing learning.

- Windows and Mac

- Level 1 CD is $195.00; online subscription starts at $49.95 a month.

Grammar Fitness
by Merit Software, www.meritsoftware.com

- This Merit program helps users to master troublesome points of grammar.

- Lessons focus on correcting errors in punctuation, proper use of tenses, and identifying and correcting errors in usage.

- Windows

- $129.00 for the professional version

My House and My Town
by Laureate Learning Systems, www.laureatelearning.com

- The client is shown a set of pictures selected by the therapist and is asked to write the names of the pictured items.

- For help, the user can copy the text or listen to the word said aloud and then compare it to see whether what he or she typed is correct.

- Windows and Mac

- For each program, the cost is $150.00 for professionals.

No-Glamour Grammar
by Carolyn LoGiudice, www.lingusystems.com

- This program includes 600 items in interactive multi-sensory customizable lessons.

- There are activities covering 10 skill areas: comparisons, have/has, do/does, copula is/are, negatives, present tense, pronouns/possessives, questions, level 1, questions, level 2, regular/irregular past tense, and regular/irregular plurals.

- Progress is recorded and reports can be generated.

- Windows and Mac

- $41.95

Paragraph Punch
by Merit Software, www.meritsoftware.com

- This Merit program helps users learn different ways to write a paragraph.

- Choosing from a menu of topics, users are guided to develop an idea and to write their own topic sentence, body, and conclusion.

- Steps include prewriting, writing, organizing, revising, rewriting, and publishing.

- Windows

- The price is $149.00 for a single user license of the professional version.

Parrot Software
by Parrot Software, www.parrotsoftware.com

- Parrot Software offers many programs to help improve writing. Some of the programs involve confrontation-naming tasks, while others focus on tasks with cognitive components, which is often more challenging. Often when clients are asked to describe solutions to problems, complete analogy tasks, or summarize written material, written expression deficits are exacerbated.

- Windows

- An online subscription is $24.95 a month for one computer.

  - **Visual Confrontation Naming** — Users are asked to type the name of each picture displayed. When they cannot recall a name, meaningful prompts are offered.

  - **Multi-Sensory Words** — An image is displayed, and the user is asked to say or write the name of it. If the "Hear Word" icon is pressed, a voice says the word. The client can choose to see the first letter of the word or the entire word written.

  - **Word Order** — This program uses a scrambled-sentence paradigm. A scrambled set of words is displayed, and the client must examine those words and construct a sentence using them. Words are selected by clicking them.

Punctuation Puzzler
by Critical Thinking Company, www.criticalthinking.com

- The users analyze context clues and apply punctuation rules to clarify the meaning of odd, convoluted, and misleading statements. The exercises are set up in a game format.

- There are different versions of this product for different age levels.

- Windows and Mac

- $59.99

WriteAssist
by Second Guess Software, www.secondguessusa.com

- **Integrated WriteAssist** is a stand-alone word-processing program, with word suggestions, spell check, and voice output for reading. Windows. $119.99

- **Universal WriteAssist** works alongside popular leading writing programs, providing word suggestions, spell check, and voice to programs such as Word, Outlook, Outlook Express, Internet Explorer, Notepad, WordPad, and ICQ. Windows. $119.99

- **C-Pen 20 by C-Pen USA, www.cpenusa.com** is helpful to move paper-based information to WriteAssist or any other program. A stroke of the pen and the printed text appears in your word processor, database interface, or spreadsheet application. PenReader reads text aloud that you have scanned using the C-Pen scanning pen. $114.95

Refer to Chapters 16 and 17 for additional suggestions regarding the use of multi-media software and many online resources with games, exercises, pictures, and adapted newspapers to improve written expression.

Software To Improve Spelling

The signs or symptoms of spelling problems may include, but are not limited to the following examples:

- Reversals and confusion of letters like *b* and *d*

- Omission of letters referred to as elisions

- Use of letters or syllables in the wrong order

- Spelling words phonetically – how they sound.

Learning to spell correctly is a difficult task to master for most children. If reading issues are present, the same underlying deficits that contribute to difficulty in reading contribute also to challenges with spelling. It is especially difficult when certain skills are weak. They include these abilities:

- Analyzing and recognizing the whole as being made up of individual parts

- Perceiving letter sounds and remember them

- Decoding written words

- Remembering sequences

Many helpful suggestions for improving spelling can be found online at http://www.ldonline.org/article/5587. In addition to these helpful tips, quite a lot of the software reviewed in this guide to help improve reading, writing, and auditory comprehension is also helpful for improving spelling.

There are a few products developed primarily for spelling help:

Title	Web Site	Price	PC	Mac	Other
I Love Spelling!	www.childrenssoftwareonline.com www.amazon.com www.academicsoftwareusa.com	$8.95	x	x	
Show Me Spelling	www.attainmentcompany.com	$129.00	x	x	

Title	Web Site	Price	PC	Mac	Other
SPELL-2 Spelling Performance Evaluation for Language & Literacy	http://learningbydesign.com	$445.00	x	x	
Spell-a-word	www.rjcooper.com	$109.00	x	x	
SpellDoctor	http://learningbydesign.com	Per year online $75.00	x		Web-based subscription
Spelling Made Easy	www.riverdeep.com www.swexpress.com www.genesis-technologies.com	$48.95	x	x	

I Love Spelling!
by DK Software sold at sites such as www. Amazon.com and www.academicsoftwareusa.com, www.childrenssoftwareonline.com

- This software was intended to be used by children ages 7-11.

- It includes interactive animated adventures that teach and test spelling.

- Players take part in an intergalactic game show adventure, playing challenging spelling games on weird and wonderful planets, and meeting their funny inhabitants.

- Games can be customized by choosing special word groups to play with—names of their favorite animals, parts of the body, country names, and more.

- Teachers and parents have access to the following resources:

  - More than 50 spelling-pattern word groups that target key spelling problem areas

  - 5,000 essential spelling words graded into three difficulty levels

  - 50 spelling-pattern word groups that target key spelling problem areas

  - More than 100 fun, themed work groups

  - Misspelled words that are automatically recycled and practiced

  - Intelligent tracking software that allows you to target difficult words

- Windows and Mac

- $8.95

Show Me Spelling
by Attainment Company, www.attainmentcompany.com

- Show Me Spelling enables people to input a spelling list or work with lists that are provided.

- 600 spelling words have corresponding speech with pictures.

- Users spell by using the standard keyboard or on-screen alphabet.

- It includes instruction and quiz modes.

- If the user gets the answer correct, various stick figures come across the screen in silly ways.

- There is a hint option the will lightly flash the next letter in the word.

- When the "show me" button is pressed, the correct spelling goes across the screen.

- Windows or Mac

- $129.00

SPELL-2 Spelling Performance Evaluation for Language & Literacy
by Learning by Design, http://learningbydesign.com

- This software program is a prescriptive assessment that identifies the precise linguistic deficits underlying each person's misspellings and offers a roadmap for providing differentiated instruction that improves spelling, reading, and writing.

- It is appropriate for grade 2 – adult.

- SPELL-2 focuses on helping professionals zero in on correcting specific problems with recommendations for word study instruction where it is most needed: These areas include

  - phonological awareness,
  - phonics,
  - vocabulary,
  - word parts and related words, and
  - mental images of words.

- Interactive characters are used during the multimedia assessment which requires minimal supervision during administration.

- The SPELL-2 software automatically adjusts to a student's abilities, providing a comprehensive assessment with detailed recommendations for differentiated instruction within 30-60 minutes (average testing time).

- Reports and letters for teachers are generated.

- Recommendations link to specific lessons and activities, connect learning needs with classroom curriculum and state standards.

- Each SPELL-2 recommendation includes corresponding lesson numbers and activities in the SPELL-Links to Reading & Writing spiral bound curriculum to provide the most appropriate instruction for each individual. This is available for an additional $249.00

- Windows and Mac

- $445.00

Spell-a-Word
by R.J. Cooper, www.rjcooper.com

- Spell-a-Word uses large print and offers built-in scanning capabilities as well as feedback for blind users.

- It is a talking spelling & keyboarding software for beginning to advanced letter users.

- This program enables parents and teachers to customize spelling lessons and incorporate spelling lists into the exercises.

- Voice prompts can be recorded and visual feedback can be used as needed. As words are learned, the verbal prompt becomes the main cue, and the visual cue fades.

- Windows and Mac

- $109.00

SpellDoctor
by Learning by Design, http://learningbydesign.com

- SpellDoctor is a Web-based writing program for Grade 5 – Adult

- It works with SPELL-Links to Reading & Writing (described above) to deliver individualized instruction and practice that transfers SPELL-Links to Reading & Writing spelling strategies and word study knowledge to students' writing.

- Working invisibly behind any Microsoft Office product, SpellDoctor automatically captures and logs all spell-checked words in a student's writing assignments, uploads them to the SpellDoctor Web site, and creates individualized Web-based instruction and practice sessions to reinforce the student's application of SPELL-Links to Reading & Writing spelling strategies in his or her authentic writing.

- Windows

- A one year subscription for one student is $75.00

Spelling Made Easy (DK)
by DK Software sold at sites such as www.riverdeep.com

- This program uses a game-show format with immediate feedback in exercises to help users become familiar with spelling rules, exceptions to the rules, and patterns.

- Strategies are taught to help develop strategies for tackling common spelling errors.

- Intelligent software assesses each student's abilities and then presents tutorial lessons for those topics where special attention is needed.

- There are over 1,750 target words.

- The program includes a special teacher's section where each student's progress report can be viewed.

- Windows and Mac

- $49.95

Software To Help Stimulate Written Content

Quite a few products are designed with activities and templates that can be used to create stories. Software of this nature facilitates writing on many topics with differentiated instruction. The templates accommodate both beginning and more advanced writers. Templates and activities are the initial steps to facilitate further strategies for writing.

Title	Web Site	Price	PC	Mac
Easy Book Deluxe	www.sunburst.com	$59.95	x	x
My Own Bookshelf 2.04	www.softtouch.com	$130.00	x	x
BuildAbility	www.attainment.com	$99.00	x	x
Find Out and Write About	www.cricksoft.com	$49.00 to $99.00	x	x

Easy Book Deluxe
by Sunburst, www.sunburst.com

- This is a book-publishing tool that provides a creative environment in which to write, design, and illustrate stories and reports.

- It includes a spell checker, a thesaurus, text-to-speech, read-aloud options, editing and formatting tools.

- The teacher's guide presents activities to introduce a variety of writing genres, with ideas and activities to integrate this program into every area of the curriculum.

- Windows and Mac

- $59.95

My Own Bookshelf 2.04
by SoftTouch, www.softtouch.com

- My Own Bookshelf provides an easy authoring interface for clinicians and teachers to create customized bookshelves for self-selected reading. It is also an effective writing tool.

- Many books ship with the software, but new ones are easily authored.

- Once a book is created, wizards are used to add images, QuickTime and AVI movies, and text. Sound options include importing, recording, or using Text-to-Speech (TTS).

- Curriculum bookshelves may also be created to support various content areas in the schools.

- With a slightly different use of the text boxes, these books may be modified for writing instead of reading. Text boxes could say "insert text here."

- Access profile for individuals can be created easily.

- Windows and Mac

- $130.00

BuildAbility (recently upgraded)
by Attainment Company, www.attainment.com

- This is a multimedia authoring program used to create high-interest books that may contain movies, text, sound, and graphics.

- With slightly modified text boxes, it also provides an opportunity for writing activities.

- Windows and Mac

- $99.00

Find Out and Write About
by Crick Software, www.cricksoft.com

- This program, which requires Clicker, enables clients to use the computer for independent research into a range of curriculum-related topics.

- Individuals read the information from the talking book and link directly to writing grids, which enable even early writers to achieve success.

- High-quality real speech gives added support on both the reading and writing activities.

- Emergent, struggling, and fluent readers can all use the resources, as the information is provided at three differentiated levels.

- At level 1, users are given short sentences that they can choose to have read to them. The writing grids, relating directly to each page, may provide sentence beginnings and endings.

- By level 3, there is in-depth information and the writing grid enables the writer to interpret and respond to the text, using the grid to scaffold their writing.

- Windows and Mac

- Prices for each CD, which provides a site license, range from $49 to $99.

Features of Word Processors and Assistive Writing Technology

Text-based and picture-based word processors and assistive writing technology can greatly improve the quality of written work. The support provided with this type of software reduces physical effort and assists with organization, so that writers are able to focus more on content. Both mainstream word processors and specialized assistive writing technology products offer a wide variety of helpful tools.

To select the most appropriate software for a particular individual, first determine which features will be most helpful to the client or student. Also, consider price and the availability of training and continued support.

Improved writing skills may be facilitated with the following features:

- Auditory feedback and text-to-speech

- Auto correct and abbreviation expansion

- Dictionary and thesaurus

- Dictation

- Editing

- Organization and outlining

- Picture/graphic support

- Speech recognition

- Compatibility with scanning pens

- Spelling and grammar assistance

- Study skills assistance

- Typing Tutorials

- Visual presentation

- Word prediction

- Web access with auditory and visual support

Text-Based Word Processing Features

Auditory Feedback and Text-to-Speech

- Auditory feedback is helpful to most writers. The computer reads text aloud after the user types a letter, word, sentence, or paragraph.

- When writers hear words or entire documents read aloud as they follow in the written text, their reading comprehension and retention as well as their written expression improve.

- The auditory feedback also helps writers maintain attention to the task, catch mistakes early to avoid lengthy editing sessions later, and improve the written formulation process.

Auto Correct and Abbreviation Expansion

- Auto correct and abbreviation expansion both correct commonly misspelled words and allow users to input abbreviations to be expanded when typed.

- For instance, if the user types "IST," the software could be programmed to expand it and type "Innovative Speech Therapy."

- Users can create frequently used words, phrases, or other standard pieces of text, saving keystrokes, and time.

Dictation

- Dictation can be used to help writers who are unable to effectively use voice recognition technology use their voice to generate printed materials.

- iDictate is a service that enables the user to dictate a document using a telephone, fax machine, or dictation device, and then receive the completed job back for editing via e-mail within a day. More information on this program can be found at www.idictate.com.

Dictionary and Thesaurus

- Many dictionaries can be customized and grammar checks tailored to the user's needs.
- Some programs read selections aloud, while others offer assistance "thinking of words" to clients with word retrieval challenges.

Editing

- All word processing programs have methods of copying, cutting and pasting, and formatting the presentation of the document.
- Some programs, such as Microsoft Word, enable users to see the changes that others make to their documents.
- The writer can decide whether to reject or accept the changes.

Organization and Outlining

- Organizing software can help people who have difficulty getting started on and organizing written projects.
- Many of these programs offer the user the ability to outline narrative prior to writing the document.
- Some of the programs, such as Microsoft Word (www.microsoft.com), do so in a linear form; others use more of a "brainstorming" technique and use webs. Draft: Builder by Don Johnston (www.donjohnston.com) provides extensive cueing and support for outlining.
- Programs such as Inspiration 8 and Kidspiration 2 by Inspiration Software (www.inspiration.com) offer graphic displays to assist with narrative organization. Each entry contains an idea, a concept, or a question that is visually linked together by branches to show their relationship to each other. Ideas don't have to be immediately formed into sentences.
- The user can have access to pictures, spell checkers, and text-to-speech. Brainstorming results can be converted into an outline and then edited to a finished product.

Picture or Graphics Support

- Many individuals with communication and cognitive deficits are unable to read and write words.

- Pictures help improve written expression.

- There are products such as Kurzweil 3000 Version 11 (www.kursweiledu.com), Clicker 5 by Crick Software (www.cricksoft.com), Kidspiration 2 by Inspiration Software (www.inpiration.com), and three programs available at www.donjohnston.com: Picture Word Power by Nancy Inman, Speaking Dynamically Pro, and Writing With Symbols 2000. In addition, dedicated communication devices such as the Lingraphica and other products by Words Plus, DynaVox Systems, and Prentke Romich enable users to express themselves by clicking on pictures to generate written messages.

- Some software and many dedicated communication devices on the market offer dynamic display. The user is initially presented with a set of pictures. Once an item is selected, more choices open up on the screen until the user finds the desired picture. A discussion of these products with dynamic display can found in Chapter 8 of this guide.

- Additional information can be researched at the following Web sites:
    - www.aacpartners.com
    - www.aacinstitute.org
    - www.abilityhub.com
    - www.ablenetinc.com
    - www.assistivetech.net
    - www.ataccess.org
    - www.closingthegap.com
    - www.rehabtool.com
    - www.ussaac.org
    - www.woodlaketechnologies.com

Speech/Voice Recognition

- With speech- or voice-recognition software and computer hardware, a user trains the computer to recognize his or her voice for writing or giving computer commands.

- This process can be used to write within a word processor or to create an e-mail message.

- The more the system is used, the better able it is to understand what the user is saying.

- Incorrect words need to be corrected by either voice or keyboard commands in order to train the program for increased accuracy.

- Speech recognition provides potential hurdles for people with disabilities—especially those with intact cognitive and communication skills who have a visual or physical deficit that prevents them from being able to type well.

- As future technological advances occur, speech recognition technology should become a more effective solution for clients with communication and cognitive issues. Products are becomingly increasingly affordable and less difficult to use.

Scanning Pens

- There are several pens on the market that scan text, including the C-Pen (www.cpen.com), Quick-Elite Pen (www.quick-pen.com), Notetaker (www.donjohnston.com), and Reading Pen (www.wizcomtech.com).

- Some of them read the text aloud, while others enable the scanned files to be sent to a computer.

Spelling and Grammar Assistance

- Different word processors offer diverse types of spelling and grammar guidance.

- Some are equipped to help typists who can produce phonetic approximations of words.

- Other programs tailor the type of grammar to be focused on during the grammar check.

Study Skills Assistance

- Almost all word processing programs offer the ability to highlight text.

- Some also enable the user to extract the highlighted material into a separate file for studying.

- Easy access to bookmarking, note-taking, summarizing, paraphrasing, and a dictionary are helpful study skill features of some word processors.

- By using the "find" feature, users can search for individual bookmarks and highlights.

- Text notes are helpful for visual processors, aiding the user to revisit and study important material.

- Using voice notes, users can dictate information such as oral summarizing and paraphrasing.

- Therapists and teachers can enter questions in voice notes or text notes, and clients can answer in either, according to their learning style.

Visual Presentation

- Most word processing programs enable the user to change the background, text color, font, and size to promote increased comprehension and retention of material.

Web Access With Visual and Auditory Support

- Several of the more advanced programs such as Scan and Read (www.readingmadeeasy), Kurzweil 3000 Version 10 (www.kurzweiledu.com), WYNN 5 (www.freedomscientific.com/LSG/), Read&Write 8 GOLD and Read&Write MAC (www.texthelp.com) offer the ability to highlight, read aloud, and extract information from the Web to other files.

Word Prediction

- Word prediction helps with many aspects of written literacy skills such as word retrieval, spelling, and sentence formation. This type of software can improve the user's attention span, confidence, independence, and language development.

- It minimizes the number of keystrokes for those with physical difficulty typing.

- The use of grammatical word prediction has been shown to improve the sentence structure and grammatical accuracy of text.

- Programs vary in the prediction methods used. Many advanced word processing programs offer the user a list of words after a letter has been typed or selected, based on previous words used. Some provide word lists based on spelling and frequency of word usage in prior documents, and phonetic approximations of words that are written.

- Some programs enable the user to select the way the words are shown to the typist and the number of words to be included in the list.

- Keep in mind that in some instances word prediction programs may actually interfere with the writing process. The word list may be distracting, and having to stop and choose words may slow down some writers.

Text-Based Word Processors

A number of word processing and assistive writing products are available to assist with the speed and effectiveness of the writing process. They differ in the features included, the level of assistive support they provide, the way they are presented, and the cost. Some products include written materials for the educator, as well as downloadable lessons with particular subject content that correlates with the school curriculum.

Try out a few assistive technology products first, so that clients can compare the usefulness and their comfort level with the features. Begin by selecting the features most important to your client, and then try a few. Sometimes the more features that are available, the better the product is for the client; in other situations, the simpler the product, the better.

There are products that work within their own word processing systems and others that work in Microsoft Word or with other formats such as e-mail or the Internet. A few products are used more in the elementary and middle school years, because they offer supportive materials that are an integral part of school curriculum. Others are geared to higher-level students and people in the working world.

Title	Web Site	Price	PC	Mac
Aurora Suite 2005	www.aurora-systems.com	$495.00	x	
Co:Writer SOLO Edition	www.donjohnston.com	$325.00	x	x
EZ Keys Version 2.50a	www.words-plus.com	$1,395.00	x	
Kurzweil 3000 for Windows Version 11	www.kurzweiledu.com	$1,495.00	x	x
Microsoft Word 2003	www.microsoft.com	$149.99	x	x
Read&Write 8 GOLD	www.texthelp.com	$645.00	x	
Read& Write MAC	www.texthelp.com	$645.00	x	
MaxWrite for Word	www.tomsnyder.com	$59.00	x	
Scan and Read	www.readingmadeeasy.com	$149.95	x	
Skeleton Key	http://www.catalaw.com/index.shtml	$99.00	x	
Talking Word Processor Version 8.0	www.readingmadeeasy.com	$89.95	x	

Title	Web Site	Price	PC	Mac
WordQ 2	www.wordq.com	$185.00	x	
Write:OutLoud Solo	www.donjohnston.com	$99.00	x	x
Solo (Co:Writer, Write:OutLoud, Draft:Builder, and Read:OutLoud)	www.donjohnston.com	$785.00	x	x
WYNN Wizard 5.1	www.freedomscientific.com/LSG/	$995.00	x	
WYNN Reader	www.freedomscientific.com/LSG/	$425.00	x	

Aurora Suite 2005
by Aurora Systems, www.aurora-systems.com

- Aurora Suite 2005 helps people with reading and writing challenges improve their writing and spelling through spoken feedback, sentence construction tips, and spelling and word selection assistance.

- It can read aloud e-mail or Web pages, menus, buttons, and text from the programs in the computer.

- The talking spell checker matches words both by visual similarity and phonetically. It can be customized to individual issues, such as confusing the visibly similar letters b, d, p, and q. The spell checker can read aloud or spell aloud any of the suggestions it makes.

- Aurora Prediction provides advanced, effective word completion and prediction that learns your writing style and it works with many different applications. It offers automatic spelling assistance, word prediction with up to 625,000 correctly spelled words in its prediction dictionaries, phonetic word completion, help for homonym confusion, grammatical prediction, screener reading, spoken typing feedback, visual highlighting for synthesized Speech, a writing monitor, and speech synthesis.

- Windows

- $495.00 for the professional edition.

Co:Writer SOLO Edition
from Don Johnston, www.donjohnston.com

- Co:Writer SOLO Edition adds word prediction, grammar, and vocabulary support capabilities to any word processor or e-mail program.

- It can be used with Write:OutLoud, which is also produced by Don Johnston, or with a program such as Microsoft Word.

- It opens up as a separate screen on the monitor and provides help with spelling, composition, and revision.

- Words are predicted based on knowledge of spelling (phonetic and dictionary), grammar rules, context clues, past written material by the writer, and letter cues.

- Struggling writers who use phonetic spelling have the special support of FlexSpell.

- The WordBank and topic dictionaries give targeted vocabulary support.

- This product is widely used in school systems to enhance many aspects of literacy.

- Windows and Mac

- $325. 00

- The newest Don Johnston title, SOLO, includes the Four Interventions: Co:Writer, Write:OutLoud, Draft:Builder, and Read:OutLoud. The cost for the bundled package is $785.00.

EZ Keys Version 2.50a
by Words+, www.words-plus.com

- EZ Keys is designed for users who have a third-grade or above reading level and cannot speak. It's also designed for speaking users who desire adapted computer access.

- It comes with dual word prediction and abbreviation expansion.

- When the beginning of a word is typed, EZ Keys displays a list of the six most frequently used words that begin with those letters. It also uses next-word prediction.

- The word prediction database can contain up to five thousand words and can be easily modified to include new vocabulary.

- Abbreviation expansion can also be used for frequently used words and phrases and for instant speech.

- The user can group phrases according to subject, such as family matters, sports, personal needs, jokes, or hobbies and then employ them quickly in everyday conversations.

- Windows

- The cost is $1,395.00

Kurzweil 3000 for Windows Version 11
by Kurzweil Educational Systems, www.kurzweiledu.com (also available at www.envisiontechnology.org)

- This program reads aloud electronic or scanned text and provides support for writing and studying with active learning, studying, and test-taking strategies.

- It simultaneously highlights and reads aloud the text with a variable rate of speech, providing the user with customizable visual tracking and auditory presentation. These features are especially helpful for people with low vision and slow auditory processing.

- The user can click on a word in the body of the text to get a definition or synonym or decode the word into syllables and spell out the letters.

- It is fluent in Spanish, French, German, Italian, and Dutch.

- Kurzweil offers both a license-to-go and remote license-to-go so that users can access the program while using a computer that is not connected to a Kurzweil 3000 Network. This option is useful for clients using Kurzweil 3000 on a home computer that cannot be brought to school.

- The Kurzweil 3000 Taskbar gives students access to Kurzweil 3000 reading, word lookup, and spell-check tools when working in other applications such as Microsoft Word.

- The Broadcast Feature lets you use the Server Administrator software to disable, enable, or leave "as is" selected Kurzweil 3000 features on multiple client computers. This makes it helpful to administer tests, protect documents, or provide consistency for user interfaces.

- An appointment calendar is included with audible reminders.

- Kurzweil can send your files to handheld devices, so you can read and reference important material when away from your home or office computer.

- This program includes a Classic Literature CD containing hundreds of titles of electronic text.

- Windows and Mac

- A single professional color version is $1,495.00.

Microsoft Word 2003 and 2007
by Microsoft Corporation, www.microsoft.com

- Microsoft Word is the standard word processing software program in both the educational world and the business world.

- It's available on both a Windows and a Macintosh platform.

- Word includes many learning and accessibility features that most users are unaware of. It is helpful to use mainstream products to promote carryover of learned strategies. Many features in this program can help clients who are struggling with reading and writing. When used in conjunction with more specialized software, it can be even more effective in helping people with a wide variety of reading and writing challenges.

- More information on Word's accessibility options can be found at www.microsoft.com/Office/system/accessibility.

- Word's spell checker falls rather short for people who have difficulty recognizing words, such as people with aphasia or visual perceptual deficits. They may struggle to read the suggestions, and without any definitions they may not understand what the words mean. Also, this program can only cope with fairly basic spelling errors, such as missing and additional letters, and very common phonetic errors. Narrator — the basic speech to text program — is not as user friendly for people who have communication and cognitive deficits, but may provide a glimpse of the client's ability to use this type of software.

- There are features included in Microsoft Word that will help the writer with the following tasks:
  - Generate summaries
  - Highlight text
  - Check spelling
  - Adjust the grammar checkers
  - Check the readability of selected text
  - Link highlighted words to dictionary definitions and a thesaurus
  - Use abbreviation expansion
  - Auto summarize
  - Adjust character and line spacing
  - De-clutter the toolbar and show only the items that are frequently used
  - Access the toolbar using the keyboard if mouse usage is difficult
  - Create templates for writing or note taking
  - Create text boxes and shapes for quick graphic organizers
  - Auto completion
  - Auto correction
  - Text-to-speech
  - Speech-to-text
  - Insert audio or text comments into documents
  - Insertion of graphics

  - Change the visual presentation of the text

  - Zoom into a portion of the page

  - Drop down option

- Windows or Mac

- Microsoft Office 2007 was released in the Spring of 2007. Most accessibility options have remained essentially the same.

- There is also a Spanish version.

- Word can be purchased bundled in the Microsoft Office Student and Teacher Edition 2003 for Windows for $149.99.

Read & Write 8 GOLD, Read & Write MAC, and Read & Write Mobile
by TextHelp, www.texthelp.com

(The products are very similar. The MAC version varies a bit from this description. Read & Write Mobile comes on a portable smart drive and allows users to run Read & Write Gold on any computer without the need for installation.)

- These products use standard Windows applications and read PDF documents.

- They use activity-specific toolbars that are stationed on top or on the side of any open application to be used as needed.

- An advanced phonetic spell checker is used to analyze and correct spellings.

- A color-coded identification of errors helps the user identify mistakes.

- They include a Spanish translator tool.

- The latest versions use the Real Speak solo voice, a more advanced scanning system, improved voice recognition, and improved dictionary.

- PDF files can also be read aloud with new hover-highlighting capabilities.

- DAISY reading technology is included.

- Read&Write GOLD allows the conversion of text to MP3, WMA, or WAV files.

- The pronunciation tutor will break words into syllables, allowing easy recognition of syllables in a word. An on-screen moving mouth will assist in the development of more accurate speech.

- These programs offer speech recognition capabilities. There are audible prompts to help with the training.

- The word prediction system learns the user's style of writing and predicts the word that's wanted next. It uses a Word Wizard, which uses a large prediction database and a thesaurus to link the writer from the words typed to the words wanted via many linking words. It also incorporates a prediction database based on a 100-million-word corpus.

- Once text and graphics have been scanned into the program, the user can edit the document.

- The Web highlighting feature allows the user to experience dual color highlighting with audible feedback in HTML documents.

- Text and images can also be scanned into Internet Explorer. This allows the user to apply "style sheets," so that preferred colors and fonts will be shown.

- The Fact Folder is a study and research tool for organizing thoughts and ideas. It captures text from any application and assists with classifying it, attaching pictures, adding bibliography information, and recording its source. When research is complete, the user can convert facts to a text document, download the text to a PDA, convert it to HTML, or turn it into a slide show.

- $645.00 for PCs and Mac versions.

MaxWrite for Word (part of Scholastic Keys)
by Tom Snyder Productions, www.tomsnyder.com

- This software provides users with a friendly interface and templates for Microsoft Word.

- It includes creativity tools not found in Microsoft Office for drawing and painting, audio recording, and converting text to speech, as well as a clip art library and prerecorded sound files and movies.

- It helps therapists and educators incorporate technology skills and enhance treatment with reading and writing.

- MaxWrite is one of three programs included in the Scholastic Keys Suite, which also includes MaxShow for PowerPoint and MaxCount for Excel.

- Windows

- The entire suite is $59.00

Scan and Read
by Premiere Assistive Technology, www.readingmadeeasy.com also at www.accessingenuity.com

- Includes all of the features of the Talking Word Processor.

- Full color or black and white scanning

- Supports 12 different languages, uses advanced settings making customization easy, and supports automatic document feeders available on high-end scanners.

- Automatic image rotation and alignment.

- Adjustable spacing for lines, words and characters.

- Magnifies up to 400%.

- Windows

- $149.95.

Skeleton Key
by CataLaw, http://www.catalaw.com/index.shtml

- An onscreen keyboard with many helpful word processing features.

- It includes a customizable on-screen keyboard, text-to-speech, word prediction, scanning cursors, abbreviation expansion, and dwell clicking.

- Windows

- $99.00

Talking Word Processor Version 8.0
by Premiere Assistive Technology, www.readingmadeeasy.com

- This program will open virtually any standard PC-based word processor file, standard text, and rich text formats.

- The Word Repeat feature repeats the word out loud after the user has typed it. This feature is used to get immediate feedback if the user has misspelled a word.

- Word Pause allows users to slow the reading of the written word without distorting the word being spoken and to increase the time between words to facilitate comprehension.

- Word Magnify highlights and magnifies words as they are spoken.

- Predictor Pro is a word prediction technology with auto learn features. It predicts the word by frequency of use and how recently it was used, as well as the content of the sentence. Generally within three characters it will predict a list of potential words for the user.

- This program can be integrated with other word processors, as well as with scanning and reading technologies. It includes twenty-two professional libraries, shorthand support, a fully customizable interface, backup and share libraries, and a built-in library manager.

- Windows

- $89.95

WordQ 2
by Quillsoft, www.wordq.com

- WordQ 2 is a software tool that can be used along with standard writing software such as Microsoft Word, WordPad, Notepad, and Outlook.

- It uses word prediction, highlighting, and auditory feedback to assist with typing and proofreading.

- When the user has completed typing a sentence, text-to-speech capabilities enable the text to be read aloud.

- The program can also be set up to read letters and words or entire documents aloud.

- Whenever the user switches applications, WordQ immediately works in that application without any additional operations.

- Additional windows are not needed with the word predictions or to read back the user's text.

- The design philosophy of WordQ was driven by advice from educators to keep it simple and not duplicate any functions typically provided by current word processors, which include spell checking, grammar checking, and auto completion.

- WordQ internally spell checks words for prediction purposes, but does not replace the spell checker. It enhances the user's spelling and grammar through its intelligent word prediction and speech feedback features, such as allowing the user to hear spelling suggestions made by Microsoft Word. This program is ideal for clients who don't need most of the features of the more complex programs.

- Windows

- $185.00

Write:OutLoud Solo
by Don Johnston, www.donjohnston.com

- Write:OutLoud is a talking word processing program that uses purposeful revision and editing tools to help writers make changes and improve their writing.

- As with other text-to-speech programs, it allows the user to hear characters, words, sentences, and paragraphs as they are typed. It also highlights the words said aloud.

- The program allows the user to use a keystroke for moving through and reading the document by sentence.

- Toolbar items can be read aloud when the mouse is hovered over the item.

- Mark for Deletion motivates users to write more, delete, and reorganize.

- The Franklin Dictionary analyzes word intent as users edit. A Homonym Checker improves homonym awareness.

- There is a feature that enables the therapist or educator to analyze the written document by word count, sentence length, number of sentences, sequential words, and number of high-level words.

- Graphics can be inserted in the text to support writing activities.

- Windows and Mac

- $99.00 if purchased alone.

- The newest Don Johnston title SOLO includes the Four Interventions: Co:Writer, Write:OutLoud, Draft:Builder, and Read:OutLoud for $785.00.

WYNN Wizard 5.1
by Freedom Scientific's Learning Systems Group,
www.freedomscientific.com/LSG/

- WYNN 5 is a multi-sensory technology that customizes content for specific learning styles and challenges.

- It provides optical character recognition (OCR), as well as the ability to scan printed pages and convert them into electronic text, and the ability to open PDF files.

- It uses color-coded toolbars with large buttons that are labeled with both pictures and words.

- The blue File Management toolbar controls the ability to scan a page and to open, close, save, and print files, as well as access the Internet.

- The green Reading Styles toolbar allows the user to customize how this software presents the document, including the font, spacing, and margins. There is also a Mask button, which "masks out" everything on the page except the section the user wishes to read. It can mask by line, sentence, or paragraph.

- The pink Study Tools toolbar offers access to a talking dictionary and a thesaurus, provides the opportunity to add a bookmark or a text or voice note to the document, and allows the user to highlight selected text using colored "markers." Words can be spelled aloud or broken into syllables. The List feature is for moving highlighted or bookmarked text into a separate document to create vocabulary lists and study guides.

- The yellow Writing Tools toolbar helps create or edit a document. The Word Prediction feature helps struggling writers and spellers. Outlines can be created and managed.

- Web Features – This software provides highlighting in various colors of text, and can track by word, line, sentence, or paragraph.

- WYNN 5 integrates its tools into the Internet, creating a clean and uncluttered page so users can manipulate reading materials.

- Users can store their favorite Web pages and view their history in WYNN's left NavBar, which makes it easier to switch between documents and read hyperlinks without activating them.

- This software also enables the user to extract highlighted text and transfer it to a separate WYNN document.

- Therapists and teachers can specify how many Web pages an individual can open while using the Internet to avoid confusion and computer malfunctioning due to too many open windows.

- WYNN blocks annoying pop-up advertisements while the user is viewing Web pages.

- Windows

- WYNN Wizard costs $995.00

WYNN Reader
by Freedom Scientific's Learning Systems Group,
www.freedomscientific.com/LSG/

- WYNN Reader includes all the features available in WYNN Wizard (described above) with the exception of OCR (or scanning) capability and the ability to open PDF files.

- Windows

- WYNN Reader costs $425.00.

Picture-based, Talking Word Processors

People with severe reading and writing deficits who are unable to use text-based word processors to write are often able to benefit from picture-based, talking word processors. These programs typically offer speech feedback, symbols or pictures to support text, and on-screen grids for writing and communication. Users create written documents by either typing directly into the word processor or by clicking on-screen grids that contain symbols, words, or letters. These programs enable the therapist to create writing activities specifically suited to individuals, incorporating as much or as little picture and sound support as needed.

Title	Web Site	Price	PC	Mac
Clicker 5	www.cricksoft.com	$199.00	x	x
Gateway Series 4: Language for Life	www.dynavoxsys.com	$2,495.00	x	
IntelliTools Classroom Suite	www.intellitools.com	$299.95	x	x
Picture Power Pack	www.slatersoftware.com	$395.00	x	x
Speaking Software for Windows	www.dynavoxsys.com	$2,495.00	x	
Picture Word Power for Speaking Dynamically Pro	www.donjohnston.com	$350.00	x	x
Writing with Symbols Version 2.5	www.mayer-johnson.com	$199.00	x	

Clicker 5
by Crick Software, www.cricksoft.com

- Clicker is a powerful and easy-to-use writing support and multimedia tool which can be used with a wide variety of clients.

- It enables the user to write with whole words, phrases, or pictures.

- Users can hear words in the Clicker Grid before writing or to proofread after writing. The words are highlighted as they are spoken.

- This software has customizable grids on the bottom half of the screen in which words and pictures are located and to which pop-up grids can be added. There is a grid-editing toolbar. Available templates include "phrases," in which an entire phrase — as opposed to individual words — is placed in a cell.

- Animation, digital recordings a variety of software voice and video can be used.

- Clicker comes with an extensive picture library of one thousand items.

- Full switch access is provided.

- Talking books can be created with a number of templates to set up books in a variety of formats.

- A very helpful support network includes access to www.learninggrids.com, which features a number of grid sets that can be accessed directly from the program. Many curriculum-based activities are available for download.

- Windows or Mac
- $199.00

Gateway Series 4: Language for Life
by Joan Bruno, www.dynavoxsys.com

- This communication software is included with many dedicated communication systems by DynaVox Technology as well as with the DynaVox Series 4 Companion and Speaking Software.

- It focuses on language development, syntactical performance, and spontaneous conversation.

- It features six distinct page sets that range from twelve to more than seventy buttons per page.

- Pre-labeled tabs containing core vocabulary for topics such as About Me, Time to Learn, Time to Play, Talk About Holidays and Time to Relax make it easy to personalize multiple pages for situation-specific conversations.

- There are more than 1,200 pages to reduce programming time while promoting higher rates of communication.

- Vocabulary is arranged by frequency of use, color coded by parts of speech, and presented in a format that allows the user to form completes sentences with less than two keystrokes per word in a consistent, left-to-right sequence. Thoughts can be quickly phrased, or rephrased, in mid-conversation using the comprehensive word morphology features and semantic power strips that the application provides.

- There are several versions targeted at different age and language abilities.

- This software is included on the Speaking Software for Windows for $2,495.

IntelliTools Classroom Suite
by Cambium Learning Group, www.intellitools.com

- This suite is a full-featured word processor that allows the user to combine graphics, text, and speech to enhance writing and communication skills using a multi-sensory environment.

- It includes word prediction; speech output of letters, words, and sentences; an on-screen keyboard with built-in scanning; a spell checker with auditory feedback; the ability to create worksheets; a graphics and sound library; and many school curriculum activities.

- This unique program allows the user to have pictures associated with their word prediction.

- Windows and Mac
- $299.95

Picture Power Pack
by Slater Software, www.slatersoftware.com

- This software provides a picture-rich environment for reading and writing.

- It includes over six thousand Literacy Support Symbols in both black-and-white and color versions. Digital images can also be added.

- When the user selects a button, the word and picture appear and the computer speaks.

- There are sixteen, thirty-six, and sixty-four Button Setups.

- The voice, rate, and pronunciation can be customized.

- This program provides picture-assisted writing so that writers can use whole words and sentences.

- Documents can be saved, and alternate modes of access, such as single-switch scanning and adapted keyboards, can be used.

- Windows and Mac

- $395.00

Speaking Software for Windows
by DynaVox Technologies, www.dynavoxsys.com

- The software that is used with the DynaVox dedicated communication devices is also sold for use on a laptop of notebook computer. Caution is given on the Web site regarding concerns about battery life, portability, and speaker quality of laptops if they are going to be used as a dedicated communication device.

- This software can assist with writing. Users can select icons and form sentences.

- DynaVox Series 4 Speaking Software includes seventeen preprogrammed communication page sets.

- Augmented communicators can access a wide range of vocabulary from a single page with the support of pop-up pages, menus, and tabs.

- Word, character, and recency prediction, along with abbreviation expansion and flexible abbreviation expansion, allow individuals challenged by significant speech impairments to express themselves rapidly.

- Windows

- $2,495.00

Word Power for Speaking Dynamically Pro
by Mayer-Johnson, www.mayerjohnson.com

- Word Power is a word-based vocabulary design that combines features of a core vocabulary, spelling, and word prediction.

- The user selects words to form messages that are read aloud by the computer. It requires a platform such as Speaking Dynamically Pro or one provided by a dedicated communication device.

- Picture Word Power enables the user to select pictures to create messages. It features written words combined with pictures to represent language and vocabulary that are organized into categories.

- Windows

- The cost is $350.00 for Word Power and $649.00 for Boardmaker and Speaking Dynamically Pro.

Writing with Symbols 2000
by Mayer-Johnson, www.mayer-johnson.com

- Writing with Symbols 2000 is a symbol-supported word processor from Widgit Software.

- This picture-based word processing program allows the user to type words with the option of having picture symbols appear with each word.

- It enables therapists to make picture materials for individuals who don't recognize text to write with pictures, and text users to have a talking word-processing program with a pictorial spell checker.

- It can be used to create resources such as symbol communication grids or for regular symbol-based word processing.

- It is also available in French or Spanish

- It includes more than 3,800 Picture Communication Symbols, each in both black and white and color, and more than 4,000 black and white Rebus symbols.

- Users can import photos or graphics and qualifiers can be added to show plurals or verb tense, adjust text, background colors and symbol sizes.

- Files can be saved as HTML documents.

- Scanning can be used with one or two switches.

- Windows

- $199.00

Stand-Alone, Word-Prediction and Word Bank Programs

The inability to recall words while writing significantly impedes the writing process. Word prediction software (a feature which was described in the previous section), word banks, and other specialized tools can be used to improve spelling, broaden vocabulary, speed up the typing process, and boost the confidence of writers. Specialized dictionaries can also be helpful for individuals with word retrieval issues. They offer a number of ways to help the writer think of words by following a series of links to related words.

Title	Web Site	Price	PC	Mac
ClozePro	www.cricksoft.com	$199.00	x	x
Gus Word Prediction	www.gusinc.com	$295.00	x	
Penfriend	www.cricksoft.com	$149.00	x	
Predictor Pro Word Prediction Technology	www.readingmadeeasy.com	$249.95	x	
SoothSayer Word Prediction Version 3.0	www.ahf-net.com	$149.00	x	
Wordbar	www.cricksoft.com	$149.00	x	

ClozePro
by Crick Software, www.cricksoft.com

- This program enables the therapist to either type in text or select text from another source such as the Internet, then select and set the remove button from the toolbar to remove certain words and leave an empty line.

- It immediately provides a fill-in-the-blank or multiple-choice activity.

- The text remains in the upper portion of the screen, minus the words that were removed.

- The words that have been removed appear in a grid of cells located at the bottom section of the screen or in sentence completion tasks.

- By clicking on the cell, the word contained in it is placed back into the selected fill-in space.

- ClozePro offers a number of options that will allow customization and increased versatility of use, including a picture library; foils that are "extra" cells containing words that will not be used in completing the activity; remove-as-you-use feature; and speech, notes, print, and accessibility options.

- The therapist can create cloze-procedure activities to be used onscreen or in a printout form.

- Windows and Mac

- $199.00

Gus Word Prediction
by Gus Communications, www.gusinc.com

- This software aids individuals with limited keyboarding ability and word retrieval deficits.

- As characters are entered, Gus Word Prediction revises the displayed "word list."

- When the desired word is seen, a click on the word or corresponding function key inserts it into the document.

- This product predicts current and next word based on frequency of use as well as abbreviation expansion.

- Windows

- $295.00

Penfriend
by Crick Software, www.cricksoft.com

- Penfriend displays a customizable prediction window directly within the word processing document.

- It has text-to-speech capability and abbreviation expansion.

- Prediction is based on first or consecutive letters typed, as well as prediction of the next most likely word based on grammar and syntax.

- Prediction improves with use by accumulating individual words for each user, creating a user profile.

- This program includes an on-screen keyboard and is compatible with many alternate computer access input modes, as well as grids produced by other Crick Software products.

- Windows

- $149.00

Predictor Pro Word Prediction Technology
by Premiere Assistive Technology, www.readingmadeeasy.com

- Predictor Pro predicts the word by both frequency of use, sentence content, and recency.

- Existing documents can be imported and this software will learn from what was already written.

- In addition to having thousands of correctly spelled words, 1,181 commonly misspelled words are included for assistance with correction. Word prediction also provides guidance with words spelled phonetically.

- A comprehensive dictionary has been integrated into the Talking Word Processor to support those who use word prediction.

- New words can be added to the dictionary, which contains about eighty thousand words. After right clicking on the word list, the definition of the highlighted word is read aloud.

- Windows

- $249.95

SoothSayer Word Prediction Version 3.0
by Applied Human Factors Inc., www.ahf-net.com

- SoothSayer Word Prediction is a software program that works in conjunction with other programs, such as off-the-shelf word processors, Web browsers, databases, and spreadsheets.

- It comes with a built-in dictionary of over eleven thousand words that can be customized.

- In addition to word prediction, it offers text-to-speech, abbreviation expansion, and sentence completion with text up to five hundred characters long.

- For speech augmentation, the built-in SoothSayer Speech Dictionary offers a foundation of over 350 frequent sentences based on abbreviation expansion that can be customized.

- Windows

- $149.00

Wordbar
by Crick Software at www.cricksoft.com

- Wordbar is displayed as a toolbar at the bottom of the screen.

- It provides point-and-click access to a variety of words, organized by tabs.

- Each tab opens a new grid with a different set of words. This essentially creates a talking word bank related to the topic tab selected.

- This program works with any Windows application that accepts text input, including word processors, spreadsheets, and databases.

- Wordbar comes with ready-made grid sets organized in five areas from school curriculum.

- Writing frameworks are given to assist with writing such as sentence starters, general words, and two blank grids for topics and phrases specific to the person's needs.

- Templates are easy to access and fully customizable. Additional templates are available for free by Internet download.

- Speech voices in many languages are available, as is the ability to record.

- Windows

- $149.00

Dictionaries

Title	Web Site	Price	PC	Mac	Other
Merriam-Webster's Collegiate Dictionary and Thesaurus	www.m-w.com	$25.00	x	x	
Merriam-Webster Online	www.m-w.com	Free (premium services also available for a fee)	x	x	Online subscription
Ultimate Talking Dictionary (UTD)	www.readingmadeeasy.com	$39.95	x		
Visual Thesaurus	www.visualthesaurus.com	$39.99	x	x	
Word Web Pro 4.5	http://wordweb.info	$19.00	x		

Merriam-Webster's Collegiate Dictionary and Thesaurus
by Fogware Publishing, available at www.m-w.com

- This dictionary offers features to search for words: by definition, by synonyms, by pictures, by origins, by audio pronunciations, words that are homophones, words that rhyme, and words that form crosswords.

- On the site, there are word games, the word of the day, and a Lookup button on the Internet browser toolbar.

- This language reference delivers information while working in word processing, composing e-mail, designing spreadsheets, browsing CDs, or surfing the Web.

- To use this dictionary, right click a word in the document, choose the Merriam-Webster icon and the definition, thesaurus, or whatever information is preset to show, and it is displayed.

- There are 225,000 entries, 115,000 audio pronunciations, 340,000 synonyms and related words, and 1,300 illustrations.

- Windows and Mac.

- $19.95

Ultimate Talking Dictionary (UTD)
by Premiere Assistive Technology, www.readingmadeeasy.com

- The Ultimate Talking Dictionary reads the definition of a word aloud and uses the word in a sentence.

- It contains over 250,000 words, including slang, jargon, and historic figures as well as a fully integrated thesaurus for referencing synonyms and antonyms of all words.

- Words are "interlinked" in many ways for cross-referencing on a variety of relational levels, so that it is easy to find a word just by knowing a concept or related idea.

- The UTD predicts the word as it is being written and presents a list of potential matches. When selected, it will read the word and its definition aloud.

- "Power searches" provide a list of all the words that contain a specified letter sequence.

- The UTD will work with virtually any program. To look up a word, the user highlights it in the current application (e.g., e-mail, word processing, Internet), presses the F11 key, and hears the definition read aloud.

- The "zoom" feature magnifies the print up to 400 percent of its original size.

- Windows

- $39.95

Visual Thesaurus
by Thinkmap, www.visualthesaurus.com

- The Visual Thesaurus is a dictionary and thesaurus with an intuitive interface to encourage exploration and learning.

- The Visual Thesaurus has more than 145,000 English words and 115,000 meanings.

- Once a word is written, the user can follow a trail of sixteen related concepts that can be read aloud.

- This program suggests spelling alternatives to help find the correct word.

- Settings and visual presentation can be controlled, as well as the types of relationships and content filtering at four different levels.

- The online edition can be accessed from any computer and is available in five languages.

- Windows or Mac

- $39.99 for the desktop edition

Word Web Pro 4.5
by Word Web Pro, http://wordweb.info

- WordWeb Pro is an international English thesaurus and dictionary for Windows.

- It can be used to look up words from almost any program, showing definitions, synonyms and related words.

- There are more than 240,000 words.

- It includes 70 000+ pronunciations, 4,900 usage examples, and has helpful spelling and sounds-like links.

- Each set of synonyms is linked to other related sets such as antonyms, parts or types, and less specific words.

- Additional features include the following abilities:

  - Solve and find anagrams

  - Suggest alternate spellings

  - Copy results to the clipboard

  - Cross-reference to other installed dictionaries and Web search engines

  - Add custom glossaries

  - Configure for American, British, Canadian, Australian or Asian English

- Option to hide (default) or flag vulgar and offensive related words
- Reverse definition (full text) search
- Cross-links words that sound the same (homonyms)
- Windows
- $19.00

Graphic Organizers: Technology for Organizing Written Narrative

For many people with writing challenges, one of the most difficult steps of the writing process is getting started. Generating ideas may not pose a problem, but recording thoughts in a clear and logical way may be difficult. Outlining, semantic webbing, graphic organizing, and visually based study software create visual-graphic support, help organize ideas, and can assist with converting those visual maps into outlines. Several programs are helpful to writers who need assistance with developing ideas, organizing, outlining, and brainstorming. Software such as Inspiration by Inspiration Software, Inc., allows users to input data in smaller segments and slowly build them into a finished document. Microsoft Word and PowerPoint can assist with organizing documents, This chapter focuses on products designed specifically to help with written organization. By using outlining software and graphic organizers, writers are often more easily able to sequence and expand their writing. With specialized study software such as RecallPlus Study Software, students can improve retention of newly learned information.

Another group of software products that help in the writing process are used to teach the development of story writing skills. These programs tend to use graphics, sound, and animation in the writing process to motivate and inspire the writer. Most are geared toward children.

Title	Web Site	Price	PC	Mac
Inspiration 8	www.inspiration.com	$69.00	x	x
Kidspiration 2.1	www.kidspiration.com	$69.00	x	x
RecallPlus Study Software	www.recallplus.com	$69.95	x	

Inspiration 8

by Inspiration Software, www.inspiration.com

- Inspiration 8 is software to help writers visualize ideas, concepts, and relationships.

- In Diagram View, writers create graphics and then analyze, compare, and evaluate information.

- The Rapid Fire tool is used to quickly brainstorm new ideas.

- More than 1 million symbols representing many words and concepts are included in Inspiration.

- Users can insert and play video and sound, such as QuickTime movies and MP3 files.

- Audio can be recorded and attached to a symbol or topic. To show relationships between ideas, symbols can be linked and words can be added to further clarify meaning.

- Users can switch between visual and outline views to further develop written material.

- The integrated Word Guide helps with word selection and a contextual spell checker automatically identifies misspelled words.

- Drag-and-drop actions and hyperlinks make it easy to gather research and connect to files and Web resources.

- Diagrams and outlines can be enriched by adding hyperlinks that connect to other documents, including Web sites, Inspiration documents, and files created in other programs. This provides an efficient way to gather research and keep work and materials together.

- This program's word processing capabilities allow writers to generate concepts and ideas and rework the document until they are satisfied. When finished writing, the user transfers the document to a word processor or onto a Web site with the Site Skeleton export tool.

- Training videos and school curriculum packets and support are included. Several versions are available.

- Windows and Mac

- The cost is $69.00 for a single user on a desktop computer.

Kidspiration 2.1

by Inspiration Software, www.kidspiration.com

- With this junior version of Inspiration, users can create graphic representations of concepts and relationships.

- Users build graphic organizers by combining pictures, text, and spoken words to represent thoughts and information.

- It can also be used as a study aid, as it aims to strengthen critical thinking, comprehension, and writing skills.

- There is a Symbol Maker drawing tool, many SuperGrouper images, and symbols paired with words in the Writing View.

- Users can add speech support by choosing to use the Listen tool.

- In Writing View, the Publish tool launches Microsoft Word, AppleWorks, or Scholastic Keys and transfers student work from Kidspiration.

- Several versions of this software are available with additional applications.

- Windows and Mac.

- A single desktop computer version is $69.00.

RecallPlus Study Software
available from www.recallplus.com

- This program is written to help with visual support for learning.

- It is a diagrammatic note-taking tool.

- Notes can be animated.

- It tracks learned knowledge and then concentrates on strengthening weak areas.

- It also gives general study tips, tracks students' revision, and gives estimates of study time needs.

- An image library is included.

- Windows.

- Expert Edition is $69.95.

Technology To Help With the Physical Aspect of Writing and Typing

The physical act of writing is problematic for many people who have fine motor coordination problems and weakness in their upper extremities. Those with mild physical difficulties may benefit from the accessibility options included with Microsoft Windows, Internet Explorer, and Microsoft Word.

Writers with severe physical difficulties may benefit from alternative input devices. These may include, but are not limited to adaptive keyboards, key guards, switches, touch screens, head-operated and eye-gaze pointing devices, Morse code input devices, brain-actuated pointing devices, voice input systems, speech-to-text software, voice-recognition or voice-command software, and cursor enlargement software. Access alternatives are discussed in Chapter 6, "Computer Access, Customization, and Hardware Selection."

An on-screen keyboard (OSK) is a visual representation of a standard keyboard that can be installed on any computer. The flexibility of the visual display combined with audio output makes some OSKs suitable for people with visual impairment as well as physical difficulties.

- **REACH Interface Author 4** by Applied Human Factors, http://ahf-net.com. Windows. $329.00.

- Additional OSKs can be found at www.gusinc.com, www.enablemart.com and www.virtual-keyboard.com.

There are a few helpful software programs that assist with typing. A comprehensive review of the many types of products available is beyond the scope of this guide. There are also a few free online programs. A few Web sites for reviewing typing software are:

- www.superkids.com/aweb/pages/reviews/typing/
- http://typing-software-review.toptenreviews.com/
- www.educational-software-directory.net/training/typing.html
- www.sense-lang.org

Custom Typing Training
by Custom Solutions, www.customtraining.com

- The keyboarding instruction can be customized to provide verbal coach-presented lessons for simple step-by-step keyboarding training.

- The keyboard graphics are very big, bright and bold, so it is very clear about which finger to use for each key.

- There are simple built-in exercises and others can be created.

- A keyboarding Goalie soccer game can run from very slow levels, so that "almost" any student, no matter how slow, can play the game.

- For users who are evaluating alternate input systems and/or specialized hardware and software, Custom Typing provides extensive tools to customize the setup which leads to the most rapid and accurate text entry.

- Windows and Mac

- A subscription for individuals is $6.00 per month.

Speech-to-Text and Voice Recognition

Several available programs will type the words that the user speaks into a microphone once the program has been "trained" to the user's word pronunciation and speech style. Most of these programs require a substantial cognitive load; several commands and sequenced steps are needed for the computer to reliably type what is said. This is often an effective method for assisting users to quickly get thoughts recorded as text, but it requires considerable practice to use efficiently. This topic was also discussed in Chapter 8, "Treatment and Technology To Improve Verbal Expression."

This type of software is difficult for clients who have communication and cognitive deficits. However, a program called SpeakQ by Quillsoft, described below, offers a potential solution for these clients.

Title	Web Site	Price	PC	Mac
Dragon Naturally Speaking 9	www.nuance.com	$199.00	x	
Microsoft Word 2007	www.microsoft.com	Home and Student Edition $149.00	x	
iListen 1.7	www.macmall.com	$99.00		x
Speak Up		Included with Mac OS		x

Dragon Naturally Speaking
by Nuance, www.nuance.com

- Naturally Speaking is a voice-recognition program that allows the user to use continuous or natural speech patterns to enter data and execute commands.

- It's compatible with many Microsoft Windows applications.

- The user can dictate directly into a PC or be productive on the go by dictating into a Nuance-certified handheld device, such as a digital recorder, Pocket PC, or Palm Tungsten.

- When synced with the PC, Dragon Naturally Speaking can then transcribe the recorded dictation.

- Naturally Speaking has a built-in text-to-speech option that allows dictated words, lines, sentences, and paragraphs to be converted to text.

- Windows

- $257.99

As mentioned earlier, this program is often difficult to use for clients with communication and cognitive deficits. It's more helpful for people with difficulty typing due to physical deficits.

iListen 1.7
by MacSpeech, www.macspeech.com

- This software offers dictation, editing, formatting, speech navigation, and voice command and Control for many applications on the Mac.

- iListen is one of the few speech-recognition options available for Macintosh users, since Dragon is Windows only.

Microsoft Word 2007
by Microsoft Corporation, www.microsoft.com

- Word includes a dictation program that can be used to determine whether a client is an appropriate candidate for more advanced voice-recognition products.

- Users can enter text, control menus, and execute commands simply by speaking into a microphone.

- The Word program is accessed by going to View, then Toolbars, and clicking on Speech. Under the Options selection, click on the Speak text button.

- Windows or Mac

- There is also a Spanish version.

- Word can be purchased bundled in the Microsoft Office Student and Teacher Edition 2003 for Windows for $149.99.

SpeakQ
by Quillsoft (www.wordq.com)

- SpeakQ by Quillsoft holds great promise for people with communication and cognitive challenges. SpeakQ was designed for those who are unable to use other speech-recognition products because they cannot fluently dictate at a fast rate, remember verbal commands, or get adequate training.

- The training part of the program is less taxing than with other voice recognition systems. Verbal models are provided for words to be repeated. This is helpful for people who can't read aloud fluently.

- There is a simpler interface than with other systems and commands are performed on the keyboard rather than having to memorize verbal directives. Speech is only used for dictation.

- Windows

- $350.00

Speak Up
by Apple, www.apple.com

- This is Apple's built-in speech recognition.

- It is difficult for people with communication and cognitive deficits to use.

SpeakQ
by Quillsoft, www.quillsoft.com

- SpeakQ enables users to dictate words into any standard Microsoft Windows document.

- Users always have a choice between typing with the keyboard, using word prediction, or speaking straight into text, while others may have Internet access, calculators, address books, text readers, a dictionary, and word prediction.

- This program is easier to train than other voice-recognition software because it will read the text to the user, and the user just has to repeat the sentence. After the software has been trained to recognize the client's speech, it can be used in therapy to practice saying utterances and try to get the computer to type what is said.

- It doesn't replace the full functionality of products such as Dragon Naturally Speaking and is not hands free.

- Windows

- $185.00

Portable Word Processors

- A portable word processor enables clients to use assistive writing technology in an affordable way.

- Some devices enable other programs to be added.

- When used in the school, consider the typing ability of the student as well as the cognitive load needed to create and open the device, handle it properly, and print the material.

- Some devices have only typing programs, while others have Internet access, calculators, and address books.

- There is a different level of writing assistance, such as the use of a dictionary/thesaurus, word prediction, text reader, and spell check.

- Storage capacity, keyboard layouts, and accessibility options vary.

Title	Web Site	Price
Dana Wireless	www.alphasmart.com	$399.00
Laser PC6	www.perfectsolutions.com	$290.00

Dana Wireless
from AlphaSmart, www.alphasmart.com

- The Dana Wireless uses Palm Operating System software in wide format, including a word processor, address book, calculator, to-do list, memo pad, and scheduler.

- Other Palm software can be added, as well as SmartApplets developed specifically for AlphaSmart products.

- There are 10 MB of memory that support over twenty thousand applications.

- Adjustable features include screen orientation, font sizes, type of keyboard, keyboard shortcuts, and sticky keys. Screen orientation and font sizes can also be changed.

- There are two expansion slots for adding memory or multimedia cards.

- There are options for Internet Access and file sharing between devices.

- $399.00

Laser PC6
from Perfect Solutions Inc., www.perfectsolutions.com

- This device provides a word processor, word prediction, spreadsheet, two telephone/databases, homework/daily calendar, scientific calculator, and typing tutor.

- It has 256K of memory and can hold forty-five named documents.

- The display can be adjusted from four to eight lines, and text and background contrast can be controlled.

- The word processor has basic editing functions and foreign language accents, and it auto saves text.

- The word prediction program can be configured to predict after one, two, or three letters, and the words can be played back with the optional text-to-speech cartridge.

- The spell checker has an eighty-thousand-word dictionary that can be accessed from the keyboard or from within the word processing program. It can be turned off for use in testing situations.

- The typing tutor has built-in exercises plus custom exercises from the word processor.

- Adjustable features include sticky keys, key repeat, and auto shutdown time.

- Files can be sent to a computer or printer using the infrared receiver.

- Optional accessories include a speech cartridge that can be heard either through a headset or through the built-in speaker. A thesaurus cartridge is available as well; however, it uses the same expansion slot as the speech cartridge.

- $290.00

Chapter 14
Treatment and Technology To Improve Cognition and Memory

Cognitive impairments in memory, reasoning, attention, judgment, and self-awareness are prominent roadblocks for functional independence and a productive lifestyle. Impaired cognition can be detrimental to rehabilitation and education efforts. The level of deficits can be severe or subtle. People with impaired cognition may display the following characteristics:

- Reduced attention and difficulty concentrating during a task

- Inability to sequence and organize information

- Poor analytical skills and judgment

- Difficulty figuring out solutions to problems

- Impaired ability to learn and remember names and events

- Inefficient time management skills

- Slow processing of new information

- Deficits planning and initiating goal-oriented behaviors

- Lack of motivation

- Limited ability to initiate activities

- Impulsive behaviors

- Faulty awareness and denial of deficit areas

Family members and clients are constantly bombarded by new information. In our fast-paced society, it's often difficult to keep up with the many demands in our lives. As a result, people with cognitive deficits may enter a downward spiral. People who experience these cognitive challenges may encounter the following problems:

- Forgetfulness following through with planned activities

- Loss of important items

- Illegible documents

- Failure to return phone calls

- Missed appointments and lack of adherence to prior commitments

- Inability to prioritize daily activities

- Disorganization at home, school, or work

Detailed information on the causes of memory and cognitive deficits and potential medically based treatments is beyond the scope of this book. However, the following Web sites provide helpful information on how memory and cognition work, types of memory and attention, diagnoses and symptoms, treatment, prevention and screening, alternative therapy, specific conditions, related issues, clinical trials, and research:

- Children and Adults with Attention Deficit/Hyperactivity Disorders (CHADD), www.chadd.org
- National Institute on Aging, www.nia.nih.gov
- National Institutes of Health, www.nlm.nih.gov/medlineplus/memory.html
- National Institute of Mental Health, www.nimh.nih.gov
- National Institute of Neurological Disorders and Stroke, www.ninds.nih.gov
- Practical Memory Institute, www.memoryzine.com

Treatment Approaches

As with communication issues, it is important to first differentially diagnose the aspects of cognition to sort out relative strengths and weaknesses. Factors that might adversely influence the client's abilities from one day to the next need to be limited. Causes may include sleep problems, depression, stress, heat, and external distractions. For many clients, a neuropsychological evaluation is helpful in which memory, problem solving, visual-spatial skills, and language skills are tested. The tests are comprehensive and will determine the individual's cognitive skills — both weak and strong.

Cognitive rehabilitation has two parts: restoring the actual cognitive skill and teaching strategies to compensate for the impaired ability. The use of state-of-the-art technology as well as strategies that do not involve technology are often needed.

Restorative Approach

- The first part of cognitive retraining — restoring skills — typically includes exercises to improve attention, concentration, memory, organization, perception, judgment, and problem-solving skills. Treatment most often uses a drill-and-practice method in which clients participate in increasingly challenging tasks. Cognitive abilities are expected to improve, much like a muscle gets stronger with increased exercise. Stimuli gradually increase in difficulty.

- A criticism of this method is that the cognitive retraining exercises are essentially artificial and have little relevance to real-world functional cognitive challenges.

- However, quite a bit of research supports the notion that appropriate practice techniques can help improve memory and cognition. The premise is that new neurological pathways are formed and improved performance enhances cognitive abilities when clients are confronted with real world challenges.

Compensatory Approach

- The second component of cognitive retraining is learning to use strategies, compensatory techniques, and tools to cope with weaker areas. Learning to use these tools not only compensates for impaired ability, but also may help rebuild the skill itself. The compensatory approach to improving memory and cognition generally focuses on the functional activities of daily living.

- Therapy might focus on helping a client remember a sequence of events to prepare for work in the morning or to complete an activity such as meal preparation.

- Look at the big picture of each person's day, and try to establish techniques, favorable environmental situations, and routines to improve the cognitive and memory abilities most needed in the client's everyday life.

- Assistive technology (AT) tools can help a person plan, organize, and keep track of responsibility.

- There are a wide variety of low-tech, mid-tech, and high-tech tools that can help clients be more independent and successful with memory and cognitively challenging tasks. Calendars, schedules, task lists, contact information, and timers can help clients manage, store, and retrieve information as well as improve time management, memory and new learning.

- More complex tools, as varied as Microsoft Outlook, Pocket PCs, and alarm watches, can also help with many aspects of cognition.

Family Support and Training

- An important part of therapy is the training and education of the client's family members and caregivers. It is vital that those who spend the most time with the client understand these cognitive strategies and encourage their use.

- The new skills and strategies that the client is learning require consistent practice.

Everyday Suggestions

- Non-tech strategies to improve everyday cognitive functioning should be tried first to help with the daily challenges.

- It is helpful to focus beyond the limits of what we see in the treatment room and talk about the specific areas in which the cognitive deficits have affected clients' lives at home, work, and school.

- Brainstorm solutions for each person's particular challenges. Suggestions may include, but are not limited to the following strategies:

  - Establish routines.

  - Organize and reduce clutter.

  - Use Calendars/daily planners, to-do lists, and phone books/contact lists.

  - Take frequent effective notes.

  - Use Web-based information management systems.

  - Minimize distractions.

  - Frequently review new information and repeat tasks to improve retention and recall.

  - Ask communication partners to slow down or repeat as needed.

  - Reduce overall stress.

  - Challenge your brain on a daily basis.

  - Break up tasks into small manageable steps.

  - Use checklists and prioritize tasks.

  - Complete one task before beginning another.

  - Take appropriate medicine as prescribed regularly.

  - Use alarms and timers.

  - Sort new information into categories.

  - Rewrite or retype information when trying to learn it.

  - Associate new information with things that you already know.

  - Ask for written summaries of information.

  - Use humor and exaggeration to help remember new information.

  - Use multiple senses when learning — write the information, say it, see it, and move in some way to help remember it.

  - Color code with colored pens, highlighters, file folders, and sticky notes.

  - Use visual aids — draw pictures and graphs.

  - Arrange items in an organized fashion, and place them in strategic, easy-to-see locations.

  - Avoid fatigue, eat nutritious meals, and exercise regularly.

- Use appropriate eye contact.

Routines

- Routines can aid memory by establishing a set series of tasks and taking the guesswork out of things.

- It's helpful for clients to keep a routine to train memory by constant repetition.

- Daily routines also help reduce stress.

Organizing and Reducing Clutter

- We are all bombarded with information. E-mail boxes fill up fast, mail overflows, belongings are placed on every flat surface around the house, and piles of things fill empty spaces. Getting organized can be an overwhelming task.

- Some families pay professional organizers to help them get started in this process. There are several associations dedicated toward establishing a more organized environment:

    - National Association of Professional Organizers, www.NAPO.net

    - Directory of Professional Organizing Consultants, www.organizeyourworld.com

- Take a step-by-step approach to helping clients and their families identify areas in their home and work environments that need improved organization. The next step is to brainstorm how to approach the situation and offer guidance for getting started.

- MyADHA.com offers an online checklist to help with school-related organization issues. It can be found at www.myadhd.com/1002areyouorganized.html. The site also offers checklists pertaining to organization of areas such as the bedroom and organizing school papers.

Calendars, To-Do lists, Phone Books, and Written Reminders

- Calendars are essential tools for all clients and caregivers, as well as professionals. They provide the most efficient means of keeping track of appointments and daily events. Choosing a calendar or planner is a very personal decision. Many clients used a system prior to the injury. Some of those systems may still work well, and others will need to be changed.

- The first decision to make when selecting a calendar is to determine how much should be seen at a time — a day, week, month, or year or a combination.

- Some clients may have been able to keep track of many things mentally prior to their injury, but now they need to develop a system to help. Children may never have developed strong organizational skills. They need to be encouraged to write down all appointments and upcoming events.

- If the task is something that may need extra effort, it can be written on a sticky note or entered into an electronic calendar several days in advance of when it must be done.

- Clients who are mobile should keep their address, phone number, emergency contact info, brief medical history, medication schedule, and names and numbers of places frequently called with them whenever they leave the house, especially if they are without their caregiver.

- In addition to helping improve organization, calendars can greatly assist with improving memory, communication, reading, and writing.

Notes

- A writing utensil and paper should be kept near all phones and throughout the living, school and work settings to jot down messages and reminders as needed.

- People can carry reminders with them and condense notes onto their calendar so that the information is kept in one central location.

- Note-taking is an essential skill for people with memory and cognitive issues. It is well known fact that by writing down information, it is more easily remembered. The notes can also be placed in strategic locations to remind people to do certain things or recall particular facts.

Web-Based Solutions for Information and Time Management

There are additional online options to help clients manage information and time.

Ta-da Lists
available at www.tadalist.com

- This is a free Web site to generate "to-do" lists. It is Web-based so can be accessed online from any computer. The My Lists page shows you your list of lists. The number of items remaining is listed, as is a note if the list is being shared with others. The dot in front of the to-do list indicates how much is left to do in a list — the bigger the dot, the more outstanding items there are. It's a quick way to gauge how much is left to get done.

Remember the Milk
available at www.rememberthemilk.com/

- This is a free Web-based task management solution. It allows the user to organize tasks into tabs and tags, and make time-specific tasks with automatic reminders and repeat intervals. It also has collaborative features.

30 Boxes
available at http://30boxes.com

- 30 Boxes is a Web-based calendar solution with a to-do list where you can add, edit, and remove tasks as well as tag them for organization.

Backpack Calendar
available at http://backpackit.com/calendar

- Multiple calendars can be created with color-coding for easy identification. Reminders can be e-mailed thirty minutes before an event, or an alert can be sent to a cell phone via a multimedia messaging service (SMS). Calendars can be shared with others.

ADD Planner
by Wolf in the Moon Software, www.addplanner.com

- This planner is designed for adults and teens with Attention Deficit Disorder (ADD). It is able to set reminders that can be spoken multiple times, appear in large print, and set to music. A tree structure is used in the Project View to help users see how projects can be broken down into branches made up of smaller tasks. A "mindfulness reminder" is used to help people become aware of their focus. $59.95

Student Life
by Tesoro Software, LLC, www.tesorosoft.com

- This planner was created to help students with attention and organizational difficulties. It can be programmed to show information about instructors, help students easily access notes, shows list of homework assignments, and categorize all the client's contacts for easy search capabilities.

- There is a social life organizer, to-do list organizer, and job schedule manager. The calendar includes a weekly and monthly view of all scheduled events with a reminder organizer. $19.95

Schedule Assistant
from AbleLink Technologies, www.ablelinktech.com

- Schedule Assistant is a multimedia, scheduling program for people who are unable to use mainstream text-based scheduling systems. Multiple appointments or events can be entered into the system by recording an audio message and designating the day(s) and time for the message to activate. A

relevant digital picture or icon can also be displayed when the message
displays. $249.00

Web-Based, Note-Taking Management systems

There are several options for taking notes and accessing them later from any
computer. They vary in their complexity and can act as effective information
management tools. Some involve typing into a text field on a page and saving it,
while others allow you to record notes to a service directly through Instant
Messaging. Some are full planners for creating documents that are more
extensive. Clients can keep a to-do or reminder list that's always visible on the
Web or it may be sent to the e-mail of others on a designated list. Notes can be
taken in school, at work, or just during the day.

Sabifoo
available at www.sabifoo.com

- This free service permits the user to post things to the Web just by sending a
  message with his or her present instant messaging account. It works with
  current IM account and software and is compatible with AOL Instant Messenger
  (www.aim.com), Jabber (www.jabber.org), MSN Messenger
  (www.messenger.msn.com), and Google Talk (www.google.com/talk./)

Backpack
available at www.backpackit.com

- There are to-do lists, notes, and images linked together as a page. New pages
  can be added. The reminder service is able to send out alerts. Rather than to
  use specific date and time, it tends to give it in terms of six minutes ago,
  yesterday, next week, one year later, which is closer to how people tend to
  think. The items in lists can be dragged up or down. With a nominal monthly
  fee, files can be uploaded and shared with others. There is no search feature.

Distractions

- It's often critical to eliminate distractions to maximize focus during tasks.

- Most clients should turn off the TV and music and avoid socializing while
  concentrating. However, some clients actually do better when there is music
  or the TV is on. For those people, trying to study in a quiet atmosphere is
  more difficult.

- Clients generally should allow the answering machine to take phone calls
  while they are actively engaged in an activity. They will be more able to focus
  on and deal with the call when they're not doing something else and the task
  at hand will be accomplished more efficiently.

- If clients are interrupted in the middle of a task, it is often helpful to write down what they were in the process of doing. This will jog their memory when they return to the task.

Repetition

- To remember information, clients need to be sure that they heard it all and processed it correctly.

- Clients should be reminded to ask the speaker to repeat information and then reiterate it to themselves to be sure that they heard what was conveyed.

- When studying it is a good idea to review the material several times in addition to using a multimodality approach, visual organization, and other helpful learning techniques.

Stress Reduction

- Many clients with memory and cognitive deficits are often stressed and tired.

- There are relaxation techniques such as meditation, massage, exercise, yoga, and general exercise to relax the mind and body.

- The level of stress is often reduced when clients make a list of the things they need to remember and accomplish, and establish a reasonable plan of action.

- The use of daily routines can also reduce stress.

Challenging Brain Exercises

- Scientists have discovered that intellectual stimulation can significantly increase the number of brain cells in crucial regions of the mind. Additional information on this topic can be found in Chapter 8, "Supportive Research."

- Activities that engage the brain and challenge it can help to keep the mind "exercised."

- Encourage clients to engage in mentally stimulating activities during the day. In addition to routines established at work or school, playing board and card games, completing crossword and jigsaw puzzles, listening to and reading books, and participating with game shows can provide enjoyment and stimulation at the same time. Additional suggestions can be found in Chapter 17, "Games and Free, Online Interactive Activities."

Small Steps

- It helps to break down seemingly overwhelming tasks into manageable pieces and do them one at a time.

- The prioritization of responsibilities and use of checklists are also useful.

Medications

- Most medications prescribed for improving memory and cognition that are currently on the market or in the process of being developed are beyond the scope of this guide. However, it is important for clients to understand what their medicines are for and what their side effects may be. Have clients research their medications on several of the sites mentioned in Chapter 19, "Online Support, Information and Discussion Groups." This activity can often be integrated into therapy sessions.

- Pill organizers can be used to help clients remember to adhere to their prescribed medication regimen.

Alarms, Timers, and Reminder Systems

- Timers and alarms can be helpful for clients to use during the day as reminders for taking medicines, leaving for appointments, and overall time management.

- Reminder systems are available in several forms such as on watches and in handheld electronic organizers.

- Alarms vary in the way they function. Alarms may vibrate, speak recorded messages, beep or display written reminders.

- Some devices can be programmed to offer many reminders throughout the day, while others may help with providing a visual display of time left for a specific activity.

Rminder.com
available at www.rminder.com

- This program sends voice and text reminders to a designated phone. The user or another person programs reminders with the specific text for the reminder, and then on the specified time and date, the recipient receives the message via voice and/or text. There is a free option that has a limit of 8 reminders a month (2 per week).

Interactive Products To Improve Memory and Cognition

There are many software programs on the market to improve cognitive functioning. They are helpful for people with documented impairments due to head injury, brain surgery, or stroke as well as children who experience attention and learning difficulties. Programs geared toward keeping the brain "fit" during the natural aging process are also becoming increasingly prevalent.

Title	Web Site	Price	PC	Mac	Other
Adventure Workshop® Preschool-1st Grade	www.learningcompany.com	$19.99	x	x	
Adventure Workshop® 1st-3rd Grade 7th Edition	www.learningcompany.com	$19.99	x	x	
Adventure Workshop™ 4th-6th Grade - 7th Edition	www.learningcompany.com	$19.99	x	x	
Arthur's Thinking Games	www.learningcompany.com	$9.99	x	x	
Attention and Memory, Volume 1	www.learningfundamentals.com	$189.00	x	x	
Attention and Memory, Volume 2	www.learningfundamentals.com	$129.00	x	x	
Big Big Brain Academy	www.bigbrainacademy.com	$19.99			Nintendo DS
Brain Age	www.brainage.com	$19.99			Nintendo DS

Title	Web Site	Price	PC	Mac	Other
Brain Fitness Program	www.positscience.com	$395.00	x		
Brain Train, Volume 1: Basic Cognitive Skills	www.braintrain.com	$129.00	x		
Brainbuilder	www.brainbuilder.com	Per month $7.95	x	x	Online subscription
Building Thinking Skills	www.criticalthinking.com	$64.99	x	x	
Categories and Words	www.bungalowsoftware.com	$149.50	x		
Challenging our Minds	www.challenging-our-minds.com	Per month $100.00	x	x	Online subscription
Clue Finders	www.learningcompany.com	$24.99	x	x	
Get Me Out OF Here!	www.criticalthinking.com	$49.99	x	x	
I SPY Treasure Hunt	www.scholastic.com	$12.95	x	x	
Memory Works	www.memoryzine.com	Each $79.95	x	x	
Mind Benders	www.criticalthinking.com	$64.99	x	x	
Moriarty Mystery Dinner	www.bungalowsoftware.com	$149.50	x		
My Brain Trainer	www.mybraintrainer.com	Per 4 months $9.95	x	x	Online subscription

Title	Web Site	Price	PC	Mac	Other
NeuroPsychOnline	www.neuopsychonline.com	Per year member- ship $425.00	x	x	Online subscription
Parrot Software	www.parrotsoftware.com	Per month $24.95	x		Online subscription
Revenge of the Logic Spiders	www.criticalthinking.com	$59.95	x	x	
SoundSmart	www.braintrain.com	Per 6 months $59.99	x	x	Online subscription
Thinkanalogy Puzzles	www.brightminds.us	$19.99	x	x	
Thinkin' Things Collection 1- School Edition	www.learningcompany.com	$69.95	x	x	
Thinkin' Things® Collection 2 - School Edition	www.learningcompany.com	$69.95	x	x	
Thinking Things Collection 3	www.learningcompany.com	$69.95	x	x	
Where in the World is Carmen Santiago: Treasures of Knowledge - School Edition	www.learningcompany.com	$69.95	x	x	

Adventure Workshop® Preschool, 1st Grade, 7th Edition
by The Learning Company at www.learningcompany.com

- These programs can build general cognitive skills as well as reading and writing.

- This bundles software includes 4 titles:

  - **Reader Rabbit Learn to Read with Phonics**

  - **Blue's Clues Treasure Hunt**

- **Arthur's Thinking Games**
- **Dora The Explorer Backpack Adventure**
- Windows and Mac
- $19.99

Adventure Workshop® 1st-3rd Grade, 7th Edition
by The Learning Company, www.learningcompany.com

- There are several different software programs that can be used to build general cognitive skills in addition to skills more directly related to school subjects.
- This bundle includes the following titles:
  - **Living Books® Stellaluna**
  - **Arthur's Math Games™**
  - **Zoombinis Logical Journey™**
  - **Kid Pix® Studio Deluxe**
- Windows and Mac
- $19.99

Adventure Workshop™ 4th-6th Grade, 7th Edition
by The Learning Company, www learningcompany.com

- There are several different software programs which can be used to build general cognitive skills in addition to skills more directly related to school subjects.
- This bundle includes the following titles:
  - **The ClueFinders Reading Adventures Ages 9-12**
  - **Mighty Math® Number Heroes®**
  - **Carmen Santiago's Great Chase Through Time™**
  - **LEGO Chess**
- Windows and Mac
- $19.99

Arthur's Thinking Games
by The Learning Company, www.learningcompany.com

- Activities build skills in patterns and sequencing, critical thinking, problem solving, memory, creativity, music, science, geography, and history.
- There are five skills levels.

- Developed for ages 4-7

- Challenges change each time they are played.

- Windows and Mac

- $9.99

Attention and Memory, Volume 1
by Learning Fundamentals, www.learningfundamentals.com

- The Orientation Module has activities for orientation, arousal, and discrimination.

- The Auditory Attention Module offers activities for sound discrimination, accessing remote memory, cross-modal matching, and sustained attention.

- The Language Attention Module includes activities for phonological processing, auditory and visual segmentation of real words, and multi-syllable segmentation of words and phrases.

- The Visual Perceptual Attention Module requires visual-perceptual matching for size, color, shape, letters, simple and complex words, patterns, and number or symbol decoding.

- The High Level Attention Module provides cognitive rehabilitation for sustained, alternating, divided, and focused attention deficits. Windows and Mac

- $189.00 for the entire Volume 1 or $99.00 for just the High Level Attention CD.

Attention and Memory, Volume 2
by Learning Fundamentals, www.learningfundamentals.com

- This software develops functional memory and attention skills by directly teaching memory strategies and then applying those memory strategies to daily living.

- It systematically targets instruction and carryover practice for the following cognitive skills:

  - Executive functions

  - Reading comprehension

  - Memory strategies

  - Visual-perceptual discrimination

  - Verbal mediation

  - Functional memory strategies

- Tasks move from simple sustained attention to alternating and divided attention with response delays and auditory distracters.

- Each exercise can be customized for specific memory needs.

- Skills addressed include basic problem solving and math, reading comprehension, inference, facts and details, and regulation of impulsivity.

- Windows and Mac.

- $129.00

Big Brain Academy
by Nintendo, www.bigbrainacademy.com

- The Nintendo DS handheld game system is used to play Big Brain Academy. It is available wherever video games and most home entertainment products are sold. Examples include Toys R Us, Best Buy, and Target.

- New users first take a five-category quiz and test their brain's ability to think, memorize, compute, analyze and identify.

- This game features 15 activities that test brain powers in areas like logic, memory, math and analysis. Up to eight people can play with a single game card, and each activity takes less than a minute to complete.

- Nintendo DS

- $19.99

Brain Age
by Nintendo, www.brainage.com

- The Nintendo DS handheld game system is used to play Brain Age. It is available wherever video games and most home entertainment products are sold. Examples include Toys R Us, Best Buy, and Target.

- There is a touch screen for writing answers with a stylus pen, and voice-recognition technology is used to identify spoken words.

- New users first take a series of tests and get a score that determines their DS brain age. Brain Age records the progression with line charts to track progress.

- This software was designed to work the user's brain with simple math-related activities and literature passages to read aloud.

- Nintendo DS

- $19.99

Brain Fitness Program
by Posit Science, www.positscience.com

- This program is comprised of six listening exercises performed on a computer.

- It consists of 40 one-hour sessions. The developers of the software suggest that users complete one session a day, five days a week, for eight weeks.

- It was developed for improving brain fitness for users.

- The Brain Fitness Channel at this Web site offers many interesting facts and research articles about memory, cognition and brain fitness.

- Windows

- $395.00 for an individual user.

Brain Train, Volume 1: Basic Cognitive Skills
by Brain Train, www.braintrain.com

- The fifty-one programs on this CD were designed to assist in the remediation of a wide range of cognitive and behavioral deficits.

- Visual-spatial deficits are addressed by programs using mazes, block designs, puzzles, visual codes and sequences, and simple to complex shapes.

- Clients can work on visual and verbal memory deficits in programs using number, letter, word, and shape sequences of varying complexity.

- Basic academic and vocational skills are developed and strengthened by programs that focus on arithmetic, spelling, reading, geography, reasoning, and typing skills.

- Time limits on many programs encourage users to work efficiently and rapidly.

- Windows

- $129.00

Brainbuilder
by Advanced Brain Technologies, www.brainbuilder.com

- BrainBuilder training was developed to improve sequential processing and advanced training in visualization and conceptualization.

- The focus exercises provide training in focus and recognition reaction time to improve concentration and response speed.

- The auditory and visual exercises provide specific training in different types of auditory and visual sequential processing.

- Windows or Mac

- $7.95 a month for online access.

Building Thinking Skills
by Critical Thinking Company, www.criticalthinking.com

- This program provides verbal and nonverbal reasoning activities to improve vocabulary, reading, writing, math, logic, and figural-spatial skills, as well as visual and auditory processing.

- Exercises involve describing characteristics, distinguishing similarities and differences, and identifying and completing sequences, classifications, and analogies.

- It is geared toward children.

- The activities are sequenced and in a game format.

- There are thirty-eight activities and over eight hundred questions with multiple levels of difficulty.

- Each skill is presented first in the concrete figural-spatial form and then in the abstract verbal form.

- Windows and Mac

- $64.99

Categories and Words
by Bungalow Software, www.bungalowsoftware.com

- This software teaches clients which words and concepts belong together.

- At the higher level, the user deduces what several objects have in common and what other objects might belong in that group.

- There are six difficulty levels. New lessons are created for each use.

- Windows

- $149.50

Challenging our Minds
by Cognitive Enhancement Systems, www.challenging-our-minds.com

- The system runs over the internet in your Web browser.

- The cognitive exercises are arranged in the domains of attention skills, executive skills, memory skills, visuospatial skills, problem solving skills, communication skills, and psychosocial skills.

- Once three consecutive passes are achieved on each of the three levels of an exercise, the user is automatically promoted to the next exercise within that domain. An assignment consists of one exercise from each domain, so there are seven exercises in every assignment.

- The system automatically keeps track of where one stops work during a session and will start back on the next session at the point where the user stopped. It is suggested that the user interact with the system 30-60 minutes a day.

- The cognitive exercises are designed as games.

- Windows and Mac.

- An individual subscription is $25.00 a month for three months. Learning Center Registration with administration interface is $100.00 a month.

Clue Finders Software
by The Learning Company, www learningcompany.com

- The ClueFinders software use mystery and adventure in their programs which are very exciting for children.

- Through interactive stories, games and exercises, problem-solving skills are developed.

- Each ClueFinders software title focuses on a specific age and skill level.

- All ClueFinders software includes detailed help features, progress reports and some add a bonus CD-ROM adventure.

- Windows or Mac

- $24.99

Get Me Out Of Here!
by Critical Thinking Company, www.criticalthinking.com

- Each activity provides an assignment, lists of one-way streets, road hazards, and tasks. The user's task is to analyze the information; use pull-down menus to choose their travel, directions, street names, places, and tasks; avoid the obstacles; and "Get outta town!"

- There are 24 activities with hints.

- This software targets grades 4-6.

- Windows and Mac

- $49.99

I SPY Treasure Hunt
by Scholastic, www.scholastic.com

- Users are challenged to select the clues in the collages; each clue helps them get closer to finding hidden treasure.

- After the clues are found, they need to be put together to get the map.

- Explore interesting places like lighthouses, train stations, and forts, while using and developing rhyming skill.

- There are many other helpful I SPY software programs that are most appropriate for children.

- Windows and Mac

- $12.95

Memory Works
by Practical Memory Institute, www.memoryzine.com

- This is a four-CD set of memory training programs to improve memory.

- The **Memory Works for Names and Faces** CD provides strategies and practice for remembering names and faces. The user learns about strategies to remember names and faces, and the program provides practice of the skills in simulated real-life experiences. $79.95

- The **Facts and Figures** CD shows strategies to help learn how to recall important facts that are already known and how to build on knowledge with new information necessary to remember later. $79.95

- The **Best Intentions** CD is designed to help people improve prospective remembering, or how to remember things they have yet to do. It shows techniques and provides practice opportunities. There is a simulation tool of a Day in a Life with items to remember and multiple distractions while engaging in various memory tasks. $79.95

- The **Nature of Memory** CD reviews the history of memory and how the brain works. It provides a self-assessment about memory and a review of external memory aids. 79.95

- Windows and Mac

Mind Benders
by Critical Thinking Company, www.criticalthinking.com

- This software offers several different levels of deductive thinking puzzles.

- Users develop the logic, reading comprehension, and mental organization skills in order to solve the puzzles and analyze each Mind Benders story and its clues, identifying logical associations between people, places, and things.

- This software is produced for middle school students.

- Windows and Mac

- $64.99

Moriarty Mystery Dinner
by Bungalow Software, www.bungalowsoftware.com

- This program works to improve cognitive, logical, and deductive reasoning skills through a nearly unlimited selection of puzzles in a wide variety of difficulty settings.

- There are many ways to customize the level of the task to meet the needs of the client.

- The visual presentation is very complex and not appropriate for individuals with visual-perceptual deficits.

- Windows

- $149.50

My Brain Trainer
developed by Cognitive Care, www.mybraintrainer.com

- MyBrainTrainer.com contains short, individual exercises designed to stimulate different parts of the brain with intense mental focus.

- The premise is that regular mental workouts of ten to twenty minutes daily can improve cognitive function and brain processing speed.

- The Basic Training program is twenty-one days. Its goal is to improve the speed of information processing and the ability to focus.

- The exercises provide immediate feedback with respect to performance (speed, accuracy, consistency, perceptual threshold), so that progress can be monitored. As brain processing speed increases, the exercises automatically become more challenging.

- Windows and Mac

- Four months for $9.95

NeuroPsychOnline
by a Division of Psychological Services Corp., www.neuopsychonline.com

- NeuroPsychOnline is a subscription-based Web site providing clinical applications for the assessment, diagnosis, and treatment of injury.

- It provides working, interactive programs and applications that run directly in the Web browser. There is no software to purchase and install. Upgrades are automatic. Subscribers have unlimited use of the software to treat an unlimited number of patients.

- This program was developed by Dr. Odie Bracy, a neuropsychologist.

- It offers six tracks of exercises that can be provided in a manual mode or an automatic therapy path.

- Categories include skills related to attention, executive function, memory, visuospatial, problem solving, and communication.

- There are fifty-three tasks with four levels of skill within each of those tasks. The tasks are arranged in the most appropriate sequence to present to clients.

- Performance is continuously assessed by the system. Clients are automatically passed up to the next level when performance reaches a certain criterion.

- Professionals can purchase a client interface subscription for home practice.

- Windows and Mac

- $425.00 for a one-year membership

Parrot Software Online program
by Parrot Software, www.parrotsoftware.com

- There are many lessons presented in a multiple-choice format with customizable levels for many of the programs.

- These Parrot Software programs, that are included in the online program, focus on memory and attention. Windows. The programs cost $24.95 a month for an online subscription.

Memory for Directions

- Either written or spoken directions are given requesting the user to move small pictures to special locations on the screen.

Hierarchical Attention Training

- Forty-eight combinations of attention activities at varying degrees of difficulty are included in the program.

- This form of treatment, where not responding is sometimes the correct response, helps curb impulsive or preservative behavior.

Memory for Animated Sequences

- An animated sequence is presented. The user then needs to select a statement about what they did or did not observe, depending on the level of difficulty.

Visual Memory

- This program presents a picture for a fixed unit of time, removes the picture, and then displays four pictures, one of which was the original picture presented.

- The user determines which of the four pictures displayed was the one that was first seen.

Word Memory and Discrimination

- This program requires users to remember a list of words and be able to discriminate the meaning between words in the list.

- Users hear a list of words and are then asked a question about one of the words.

Word Recognition

- Users must remember a list of two to ten words. Then, when words are displayed one at a time, users must determine whether the displayed word is a member of the list.

Auditory and Visual Instructions

- Four geometric forms are displayed. A description of one of the geometric forms is then presented using the attributes of size, color, and shape (e.g., large, yellow, square).

- The user must identify the geometric form that fits the description.

Compensatory Memory Strategies: Chunking

- Memory of large bodies of information is facilitated by dividing the information into smaller, related chunks of information.

- The components of a chunk of information can be related by category, color, size texture, function, or definition.

Revenge of the Logic Spiders
by Critical Thinking Company at www.criticalthinking.com

- Each activity was produced to sharpen reasoning and comprehension through multiple-choice word problems that become progressively more challenging. Each possible answer must be read and analyzed carefully. Only the correct inferences and deductions allow students to escape the hungry spiders.

- There are 116 logic problems and three maze sizes.

- Targeted for 6-12th grade.

- Windows and Mac

- $59.95

SoundSmart
by Brain Train, www.braintrain.com

- This program uses game-like brain-training exercises designed to help improve phonemic awareness, listening skills, working memory, mental processing speed, and self-control.

- Attention Coach is offered with three levels of difficulty. Spoken instructions become increasingly complex as the user progress through alphabet games.

- Math and Memory Coach is offered with multiple skill levels. Users are presented with math problems to perform mentally. The player must wait to answer until the stoplight turns green. Sometimes it delays on the yellow light, then changes its mind altogether about the question. When questions are answered correctly, parts of pictures are uncovered.

- Sound Discrimination Coach offers three levels of difficulty. Users are given phonemic awareness drills to improve listening skills under many types of conditions.

- SoundSmart offers three behavioral tracks to access the tasks within each program and customize them as needed. They are the Speed Track, Patience Track, Listening Track, and Challenge Track.

- Windows and Mac

- $59.00 for a 6 month lease.

Thinkanalogy Puzzles
by Critical Thinking Company, www.brightminds.us

- This program builds vocabulary and reading comprehension skills with the use of analogies.

- In each activity, users analyze thirty potential analogy pairs, evaluate word meanings and relationships to find the best matches, and then classify each analogy by type.

- There are twenty exercises with three hundred analogies.

- Windows and Mac

- $19.99

Thinkin' Things Collection 1, School Edition
by The Learning Company at www.learningcompany.com

- Developed for ages 3-7.

- Improves visual and auditory memory
- Builds logical, musical, spatial, and kinesthetic thinking skills
- Provides opportunity to compare and contrast attributes
- Enhances observation and perception abilities
- Introduces hypotheses and testing of rules
- Introduces the relationship between scientific exploration and creativity
- Windows and Mac.
- $69.95

Thinkin' Things® Collection 2, School Edition
by The Learning Company at www.learningcompany.com

- Developed for ages 7-11.
- Five activities are included that help students explore their musical and artistic abilities as well as strengthen their memory, visual and spatial awareness, listening and problem solving skills.
- Windows and Mac
- $69.95

Thinking Things Collection 3, School Edition
by The Learning Company at www.learningcompany.com

- Developed for ages 8-14.
- Introduces and reinforces deductive reasoning, logic, observation, visual analysis, creativity, basic elements of computer programming and problem solving
- Strengthens pattern and sequence recognition as well as finding multiple solutions to problems
- Windows and Mac
- $69.95

Where in the World is Carmen Santiago: Treasures of Knowledge, School Edition
by The Learning Company, www.learningcompany.com

- This program is suitable for ages 8 and older.

- Players improve their world geography and problem-solving skills while tackling challenging missions, solving mind-bending puzzles, and uncovering stolen treasures.

- Expands knowledge of geography, cultures and landmarks of 50 different countries

- Encourages close observation and deductive reasoning

- Develops skills in decision making, listening and following directions, data collection, database research and map reading

- Builds critical thinking and problem-solving skills

- Supports state and national social studies standards

- Windows and Mac

- $69.95

Cue Card 1.5
by Wade Brainerd
www.download.com/3000-2051-10075304.html

- Free Electronic Flash Card Tool

- Users decide what to work on and CueCard will quiz the user on them.

- CueCard features smart testing, which automatically focuses on the items that are the most difficult.

- It offers printing (including custom page layouts and sizes), pictures and sounds on cards, Unicode support, card formatting, a multi-lingual user interface, Import/Export, a study time.

- Free

Study Stack
by John Weidner, www.studystack.com

- This is a free, online program that can be used to access already included study stacks or make customized stacks.

- A stack of "virtual cards" contain information about a certain subject.

- Users review the information, discarding the cards that were already learned and keeping the others for additional review.

- Each card can show multiple pieces of information; and the whole stack can be automatically sorted by any one of the pieces of information.

- The data for a studystack can be displayed as flashcards, a matching game, a word search puzzle, and a hangman game.

- The information can be exported to smart phones and PDAs.

- Free

Assistive Reading and Writing Software

Clients who have cognitive and memory challenges most often have difficulty with reading and writing. They may lose their train of thought while writing, have difficulty sequencing sentences into a coherent paragraph, require extensive editing of written documents, and lack retention of information that they read. A wide range of tools is available to help with many aspects of reading and writing.

Please refer to Chapters 12 and 13 for assistive reading and writing technologies.

Devices To Assist With Memory and Cognition

A number of tools and devices are available to help with memory, organization, time management, and executive functioning skills.

Digital Recorders

- Digital recorders make excellent assistive aids.

- The battery life, compact size, and amount of audio storage have improved greatly in the past few years.

- Files can be copied to a CD as WAV files or converted to text with advanced voice-recognition software.

- The unit can play reminders and instructions at preset times.

- Digital recorders can also function to supplement a person's memory. The user can record and listen to the ideas and reminders later on.

- PDAs, smart phones, and MP3 players such as iPods also have many of these capabilities.

For more information, refer to these Web sites:

- www.olympusamerica.com
- www.next-wave-solutions.com

Electronic Organizers

- An electronic organizer is a personal information management tool. There are many varieties ranging from simple to complex. They all include a calendar or schedule planner, an address book with contact information, a calculator, and a clock that may have an alarm. The introduction of such a system improves the client's ability to establish daily priorities, follow through with planned activities, recall events of the past, and prepare for the future.

- The most basic systems generally have small buttons, are black and white, have small screens, don't offer PC connectivity, and accept data only via the keyboard. Electronic organizers are often difficult for people with dexterity and cognitive limitations to use. If these items are lost, there is generally no backup with the information.

- More advanced organizers (generally referred to as Personal Digital Assistants, or PDAs) or handhelds are built on a Palm or Pocket PC platform. Many of their advanced features are helpful for people with communication and cognitive deficits. Some of these features include wireless access, the ability to use other handheld software, the ability to synchronize the information to a computer, and accessibility features such as text readers and voice recognition.

- PDAs can also offer software applications such as spell checkers, advanced scheduling software that integrates notes and reminders, Internet access, e-mail programs, and photo albums. These features reduce the demands on working memory and can provide practical solutions to everyday issues when programmed well; however, clinicians need to be sure that clients do not become overly dependent on them, or confused or distracted by them.

The following Web sites may be helpful in the search for these devices:

- www.dell.com
- www.franklin.com
- www.microsoft.com/mobile/pocketpc
- www.palm.com

Handheld Devices Produced for Clients With Cognitive Challenges

In addition to the mainstream electronic organizers and PDAs described above, there are devices that have been produced for people who may need additional support with memory, organization, and daily routines. They generally offer an interface that is more user-friendly and that is structured to meet the needs of people with communication and cognitive challenges. Phone support is most often provided for programming.

Community Integration Suite
by AbleLink Technologies, www.ablelinktech.com

- The Community Integration Suite comes ready to go with a Pocket PC, Pocket Compass (picture/audio-based prompting/cueing application), Schedule Assistant (time-based audiovisual cuing), and Discovery Desktop (a custom Windows desktop).

- The computer automatically turns on and cues the user to begin a task, travel to a specific location, or remember an event or appointment.

- It offers time-based cues with specific instructions.

- Caregivers set up the various daily, weekly, and monthly tasks and time cues with audio and custom pictures on the computer.

- $1,499.00 for the entire system

Loc8tor
from Loc8tor, Ltd., www.loc8tor.com

- Loc8tor helps find important possessions with the use of a homing device.

- In the Locate mode audio beeps and the on-screen directional display guide users quickly and easily to mislaid tagged items.

- In the Alert mode an invisible safety zone can be established around the Loc8tor (plus) alerting the user with audio-visual and vibration alarms should tagged items move out of the set boundary.

- Small, discrete tags and a compact handheld unit direct users from up to 183 meters / 600 feet to within 2.5cm / 1" of the mislaid item.

- $99.99

VoiceCue
available from Attainment Company, www.attainmentcompany.com

- This is an auditory cueing device that holds up to five messages for a total of sixty seconds of recording time.

- A message can be recorded and the clock set to play it at a preset time.

- Each message can be assigned two playback times.

- A replay feature allows messages to be repeated within one minute.

- $39.00

Chapter 15:
Adapted E-mail, Search Engines, and Web Browsers

The Internet has changed the way many of us carry out everyday social, vocational, and leisure pursuits. It has become an integral part of our lives that permits us to take advantage of a wide range of tasks in an efficient and convenient way. Use of e-mail and the Internet can help link people with community, friends, and family. Online access provides a way to efficiently gather information.

The ability to use the Internet and e-mail is especially important for people with communication and cognitive deficits for a number of reasons. It offers

- a means of communication for people who have difficulty talking,

- a written record of communication for people with memory issues,

- a practical, meaningful way to practice functional reading and writing skills,

- easier access to information, and

- an efficient way to plan and coordinate activities.

Many people with communication and cognitive challenges never try or initially fail with their attempts to use e-mail, instant messaging (IM), and listserv or chat room discussions. However, with the use of helpful tools and strategies, many people can successfully use these forms of communication.

In addition to the assistive reading and writing tools reviewed in prior chapters, adapted e-mail programs and specialized Web browsers that can assist with successful Internet use can also benefit clients.

Strategies To Use With Already Established E-mail Accounts

- Produce printed communication sheets with tailored greetings, questions, and descriptions of daily activities which the user would send. The client can then copy these sentences into the e-mail. The written information acts as a "social script" for communication. Templates are also useful.

- Develop designated files on the client's computer that contain questions and sentences to cut and paste for use in e-mail messages.

- Load a talking program such as WordQ or Universal Reader that will speak the messages aloud as the client types them. The auditory feedback often makes errors more noticeable at the time they are produced, which reduces the amount of editing that needs to be done at the end.

- Use word prediction software, a thesaurus or a dictionary with relational links for people with word retrieval deficits to use while typing messages. These suggestions were discussed in Chapter 13, "Treatment and Technology to Improve Written Expression."

- Use a talking word processor that is compatible with e-mail to facilitate reading and writing. These suggestions were also discussed in Chapter 13 of this guide.

- Configure the existing e-mail account if possible to make it more user-friendly. Most have help features to describe options for changing the font (such as by making it larger) and the number of steps in the sequence. Settings may allow users to automatically enter the password, read the next e-mail, and check the spelling.

Adapted E-mail Programs

As with other types of programs, adapted e-mail programs offer different features. They may include the following features:

- The ability to send a message using recorded voice.

- The ability to send messages by selection of pictures to communicate a message.

- The use of pictures in the address book.

- A simplified user interface.

- Text-to-speech technology, which reads aloud incoming messages.

- Speech recognition engines, so that spoken messages used to write the messages are converted to text as well as sent as a sound file attachment.

- Simplification of sequencing of steps with spoken and visual prompts.

- Self-contained e-mail groups.

- Inclusion of training programs to learn to use the software.

- Inclusion of video messages.

E-mail Using Recorded Voice

Many people who are unable to read or write, but can speak intelligibly may benefit from voice-based, e-mail systems. E-mail that uses recorded voice can enable AAC users to send audio e-mail using their communication device. In addition to using the programs mentioned below, people may use voice recognition technology such as Speak Q, described in Chapter 13 of this guide.

Title	Web Site	Price	PC	Mac	Other
Coglink E-mail	www.coglink.com	$10.00	x		Online subscription
ICanEmail	www.rjcooper.com	$109.00	x	x	
Springdoo	www.springdoo.com	Free	x	x	Online
Talking Aide Wireless	www.zygo-use.com	$5,995.00			Device
V3 Mail	www.V3Mail.com	Free	x		
VeMail	www.vemail.com	Free	x		
Web Trek Connect	www.ablelinktech.com	$249.00	x		
YackPack	www.yackpack.com	Free	x	x	

Coglink E-mail
by Think and Link at www.coglink.com

- This is a personalized, simple-to-use e-mail program designed for individuals with significant cognitive impairments.

- It helps users build their own community of e-mail buddies. Only people on the correspondent list managed by the help desk can exchange messages.

- Users are protected from junk e-mail and viruses through the Coglink program.

- Coglink includes an automated training program that helps users learn all the basic kills for using the mouse, keyboard, and e-mail.

- Windows

- $10.00 a month.

IcanEmail
by RJ Cooper at www.rjcooper.com

- This is a full-screen, talking e-mail program designed with a basic interface for users with cognitive, visual, and/or physical challenges.

- The program asks a series of questions, one at a time to help the user sequence the steps.

- The user can speak messages, and the recorded voice is sent.

- If using AOL, a program called IzzyMail (www.pop3hot.com) will also need to be installed.

- The e-mail "partner" (the sender or recipient) can send and receive mail without any special software.

- Windows and Mac

- $109.00.

Springdoo
by Springdoo at www.springdoo.com

- This enables users to speak into a microphone and send videos by e-mail.

- The recipient of the video message clicks on a link to watch and listen to the message, and then can reply to the message.

- It can be sent along with a text message, so that the user can decide whether to read the text or listen to the audio.

- Windows or Mac

- Free

TalkingAide Wireless
by Zygo Industries at www.zygo-use.com

- The TalkingAide Wireless is a text-to-speech device designed specifically for cell phone and e-mail use.

- It uses speech synthesis with seven voices.

- It offers a normal typing mode (up to 20,000 characters) and a chat mode for writing and engaging in secondary conversations.

- There are function keys for easy selection of onscreen options such as word completion predictions.

- There is a 6" display with backlighting and 3 font sizes.

- This rugged device weighs 3.5 pounds and is 10.5 x 8.75x3 inches.

- $5,995.00

V3 Mail
by V3Mail at www.V3Mail.com

- V3 mail is an Internet program designed for PCs that makes it easy to create and send voice and video e-mail messages.

- This software offers voice messages (MP3) as well as translation of written messages to speech using text to speech technology.

- Windows

- There is a free version or a pro version with additional features such as no advertising for $39.99.

Vemail
by NCH Swift Sound at www.vemail.com

- This software allows the user to use ordinary e-mail to record a message instead of typing it. The F6 key is depressed while speaking. The message is compressed and sent as an attachment.

- Anyone can receive and listen to the Vemail. It can be played with the standard player installed in almost all computers.

- If a speech recognition engine is installed on the sender's computer, it will translate the recording into text and include it with the e-mail.

- This program can also be used to send and receive e-mail with a cell phone for $4.99 a month.

- Messages can be read using text-to-speech software and replied to with voice.

- Free

Web Trek Connect
by AbleLink Technologies at www.ablelinktech.com

- This program provides a simplified picture-based system for both receiving and sending e-mail with standard e-mail programs. It uses photos and spoken prompts to guide the user through selecting an e-mail address, recording a spoken message, then sending the message.

- When receiving mail, the user needs only to click on the sender's picture to initiate the built-in screen reader or to automatically play an attached audio recording. The user's e-mailbox can be set up so that it receives messages only from people in the address book.

- Windows

- This program is part of the Computer & Web Access Suite, but can be purchased separately for $249.00.

YackPack
by YackPack at www.yackpack.com

- YackPack allows users to create online voice messages and share those messages with private or public groups.

- Windows or Mac

- There is a free version, as well as options with more features.

E-mail Using Pictures To Compose Messages

Many clients would like to send e-mail messages, but are unable to write or copy messages or to speak clearly. One potential adaptation would be to send messages that use pictures rather than words. Unfortunately, there are no ideal solutions that enable someone to compose messages with pictures and send them directly in e-mail. Mayer Johnson used to produce a product called Inter_Comm, but it has been discontinued.

Currently the best alternative for helping clients use e-mail to send messages is to formulate text messages with communication devices or with picture-based word processors. Text can be saved into a file that can be copied into the e-mail.

Adapted Search Engines and Web Browsers

Many Web pages and search engines are too complex for users with communication and cognitive challenges. People with visual impairments or reading difficulties can benefit from special browsers or customizing a mainstream browser to make them easier to see and use. Some offer text-to-speech, speech recognition, or alternate access modes.

Title	Web Site	Price
Firefox	www.mozilla.org	Free
Internet Explorer 7	www.microsoft.com	Free
Kartoo	www.kartoo.com	Free
Speegle	www.speegle.co.uk	Free
Web Trek	www.ablelinktech.com	$249.00

Firefox
by Mozilla at www.mozilla.com

- Firefox is a free Web browser that comes with many built-in features for customization through free add-ons.
- Access Firefox at www.accessfirefox.com/index.html presents and showcases the accessibility tools and features that are available.

- Firefox is available for Windows, Mac, and Linux. It is also available in different languages.

Internet Explorer 7
by Microsoft Corporation at www.microsoft.com

- Internet Explorer is a popular Web browser that offers quite a few accessibility options that allow it to be configured for improved display and readability.

- Accommodations can be selected to make the keyboard and mouse faster and easier to use, zoom in on a Web page, change Web page colors, font and text size, and format pages with a style sheets.

- More information can be found at http://www.microsoft.com/enable/products/IE7/default.aspx.

- Free

Kartoo
by Kartoo Technologies, at www.kartoo.com

- Kartoo is a Meta search engine which presents its results on a map.

- After a word to search for is typed, Kartoo analyzes the request, questions the most relevant engines, selects the best sites and places them on a map.

- This site is offered in eight languages. It uses Flash technology to display the interactive maps, but there is also an HTML version available.

- The Web sites are mapped as balls with the largest ball containing the most relevant information. When the pointer is passed over the balls, a description of the site is displayed. By moving the mouse over the topics on the map, the user can see the relationship between the topic and the search terms.

- If the topic is very relevant, the user can click the plus sign to add it to the search term or click minus to remove it from the map.

- A series of keywords appears. You can refine your search by clicking subjects.

- Free

Speegle
by CEC Systems, www.speegle.co.uk

- A speech technology company that delivers Google search results as speech.

- Free

Web Trek
by AbleLink Technologies at www.ablelinktech.com

- Web Trek is a picture-based browser that allows the user to capture a picture directly off of a Web page and displays the picture as a large button on the main Web Trek page.

- The Web site can then be accessed by clicking on the picture. Once the Web site is accessed, the site is navigated through its traditional link buttons.

- Large arrows are displayed for moving to the next or previous page.

- If the symbol mode is selected, the text is presented in a simplified display with symbols above the words; the user still sees the graphics on the site.

- Text mode presents the same simplified display without the symbols, although still including the graphics.

- The text can be converted to a preferred font which is easier to see and can be read aloud. The program speaks sentence by sentence, highlighting each word as it is spoken.

- Links can be spoken before they are selected. Webwide provides symbol support for text on Web pages using Widgit Rebus symbols described at (www.widgit.com.)

- $249.00

Web Trek is part of the **Computer & Web Access Suite,** which includes Web Trek Connect (described above) and Discovery Desktop, a custom Windows desktop. The cost for the suite is $299.00.

Chapter 16:
Multi-Media Programs and Generating Printed Treatment Materials

Programs that generate treatment material and others that provide interactive use of recordings, drawing, graphics and other features that provide the ability to manipulate and create novel products have emerged as resources from which to obtain effective and affordable materials to use in treatment. These powerful technological tools have become mainstream in many educational, business, and home settings. Clip art, digital photos, and recordings can be used to customize worksheets, games, calendars, communication aids, and interactive talking books. These products lend themselves particularly well to treatment that addresses multiple goal areas.

The benefits of using products to generate therapy materials that provide the ability to manipulate sound, graphics, and voice are many:

- They save time by providing ready to use materials.

- They minimize the need for additional purchases.

- They provide interesting, fun and new treatment presentation formats.

- They may provide relevant customized stimuli.

Programs To Produce Customized Therapy Materials To Print

There are several programs that can be purchased to generate customized written materials that can be used either during treatment sessions or later by a client during independent practice. With easy access to these programs and a printer, there is less reliance on workbooks and other treatment materials.

Title	Web Site	Price	PC	Mac	Other
40,000 Selected Words CD	www.harcourtassessment.com	$49.00	x		
Edhelper.com	www.edhelper.com	Per year $19.99	x	x	Online subscription
FreeForm Speech Therapy Worksheets	www.bungalowsoftware.com	$69.50	x		

Title	Web Site	Price	PC	Mac	Other
Speaking Of Speech CD v.1	www.speakingofspeech.com	PDF on CD $25.00	c	c	
Therasimplicity	www.therasimplicity.com	Per year $249.99	x	x	Online subscription

40,000 Selected Words CD
by Harcourt Assessment, www.harcourtassessment.com

- This CD enables the user to search for words according to the phonemes, syllable length, and position of the sound that are needed.

- *40,000 Selected Words* includes the full phonetic spelling of each word and lists them in alphabetical order to enable the clinician to quickly develop custom lists to practice target sounds with clients.

- Windows

- $49.00

Edhelper.com
by Edhelper.com, www.edhelper.com

- This online subscription is geared toward helping professionals who work with elementary age students.

- Personalized crossword puzzles, quizzes, worksheets and thematic activities can be created based on specific grade level and other variables.

- Windows and Mac

- $19.99 a year.

FreeForm Speech Therapy Worksheets
by Bungalow Software, www.bungalowsoftware.com

- This software enables users to print customized worksheets or provides clients with an opportunity to work directly on the computer.

- The font style and size can be selected, and lessons can be customized according to the communication modality and level of practice.

- Topics include auditory comprehension, verbal expression, reading, writing, articulation, oral-motor, swallowing, and cognition.

- Windows

- $69.50

Speaking Of Speech CD v.1
by Speakingofspeech.com, www.speakingofspeech.com

- This CD offers many communicating-building activities for speech pathologists and teachers.

- Many of the materials are made with Boardmaker symbols and are appropriate for students in regular and special education.

- The CD includes:

  - Extension activities for 25 children's books

  - Phonemic awareness activities

  - One-Minute Drills for phonemic practice in the classroom

  - Games on the Go and Reading Tips for parents

  - Posters, games, and spinners for articulation and language

  - Summer speech/language activity packet

  - Year-round activity pages for counting and graphing

  - Caseload management materials (sticker chart, homework magnets, speech passes)

  - Communication boards for AAC/inclusion students

  - Handouts, parent questionnaires, and info sheets for AAC, switch use, functional communication, vocational training, and community-based instruction

- PDF file format for Windows and Mac

- $25.00

Therasimplicity
by Therasimplicity, www.therasimplicity.com

- Therasimplicity is an online library of over 1,200 customizable tools for therapy.

- Materials can be printed or used at the computer with a client.

- The program includes an extensive collection of worksheets, pictures, illustrations, flashcards, exercises, and games. There are over 1,100 images.

- The program is continually expanded and improved.

- Materials are provided for:

  - Articulation and phonology

  - Fluency

- Voice and resonance
- Receptive and expressive language
- Hearing
- Swallowing
- Cognition
- Social communication
- The online library is Web-based and accessible from any computer with online access.
- Windows and Mac
- An annual subscription is $189.99.

Online Free Non-Interactive Treatment Materials

Many Web sites offer free materials that can either be printed out to use in therapy, or used directly on the computer. Word lists and sentences produced for particular treatment tasks save time and expense.

The following sites are very helpful in therapy for functional phrases and sentences, articulation drill and practice lists or auditory stimulation materials:

AAC messaging and vocabulary lists
available at http://aac.unl.edu/vbstudy.html

- This site offers targeted vocabulary lists. There are high-frequency word lists for preschool, school age, and young adults.
- List of functional phrases are also provided for small talk for children and adults, context-specific messages, and vocabulary for school settings.

English and Spanish articulation and language exercises to download
available at www.aphasianyc.org

- This site by AphasiaNYC.org provides many free speech and language printouts in both English and Spanish.
- Click on "therapy resources." The materials were produced to help people with aphasia, but can be used to help many types of clients.

Internet Training Package for people with aphasia
available at www.shrs.uq.edu.au/cdaru/aphasiagroups/index.html

- The University of Queensland Aphasia Group produced this site for people with a communication or literacy disability.

Resources for Clinicians
available at web.utk.edu/~pflipsen/Clinical_Resources.html – provided by Peter Flipsen

- This site includes three sections:
  - A decision tree to help sort out trouble separating out articulation (phonetic) problems from phonological (phonemic) problems in children
  - A speech perception test
  - Listening lists for auditory bombardment

The SLP Start Page
by Caroline Bowen, http://www.speech-language-therapy.com/slp-eureka.htm

- Type "minimal pairs" in the search box to access free phonology and articulation resources.

PuzzleMaker
available at http://puzzlemaker.school.discovery.com/

- Puzzlemaker is a puzzle generation tool for teachers, students and parents.
- This online site enables users to create and print customized word search, crossword and math puzzles using your word lists.

Worksheets Unlimited
available at http://worksheetsunlimited.org

- This site offers free downloads of worksheets for many easy lessons, flash cards, printable calendars, awards, certificates, maps, coloring pages, phonics rules, phonics worksheets, list of Dolch site words, handwriting worksheets in five fonts, printable games, charts, and chore card.
- There is a message board for educators.
- 100 lessons, theme units, and many curriculum ideas are provided.

Multi-Media Interactive Authoring Programs

Most of these products are very engaging and can be used to target multiple treatment goals. They work best with creative therapists who tailor the programs to match the needs of each user to stimulate interest. These products are more appropriate to use during 1:1 sessions and not as part of individualized practice programs.

Many of these tools can be used to create symbol-based print and interactive materials such as story boards, talking books, communication displays, visual schedules, symbol-supported literacy activities, worksheets, writing activities, and activities to promote general educational and functional living skills.

Title	Web Site	Price	PC	Mac	Other
Boardmaker Plus!	www.mayerjohnson.com	$539.00	x		
BuildAbility	www.donjohnston.com	$99.00	x	x	
Clicker 5	www.cricksoft.com	$199.00	x	x	
Online Greeting Cards	www.bluemountain.com www.123greetings.com www.americangreetings.com www.hallmark.com.	Free	x	x	Online
HyperStudio 4.5	www.sunburst.com	$69.95	x	x	
Kidspiration 2.1	www.inspiration.com	$69.00	x	x	
IntelliPics Studio 3	www.intellitools.com	$139.95	x	x	
KidPix Deluxe 4	www.broderbund.com	$34.99	x	x	
Photo Story 3	www.microsoft.com	Free	x		Free download
Pixie	www.tech4learning.com	$44.95	x	x	
PowerPoint 2003 and 2007	www.microsoft.com	$219.99	x	x	
WebBlender	www.tech4learning.com	$44.95	x	x	

Boardmaker Plus!
by Mayer-Johnson, www.mayerjohnson.com

- Boardmaker Plus! adds the interactivity of voice, animations, and video capability to Boardmaker.

- Featuring more than 4,500 Picture Communication Symbols (PCS) in both color and black-and-white, all in 44 languages, Boardmaker Plus! is a drawing program combined with a graphics database that also has the ability to talk and play recorded sounds and movies.

- A new feature referred to as the Symbolate button enables the user to type and symbols appear.

- Boardmaker Plus! Includes more than 150 sample interactive boards and more than 100 interactive templates.

- Windows
- $539.00

BuildAbility
by Don Johnston, www.donjohnston.com

- BuildAbility is an authoring tool for building single-switch, early literacy activities and lessons.
- A multimedia page can be produced by using a one-click toolbar to select or draw a picture, add text and sound, and select page advancement.
- Literacy activities created by Caroline Musselwhite, Patti Rea, and other literacy experts are included.
- Windows and Mac
- $99.00

Clicker 5
by Crick Software, www.cricksoft.com

- Clicker 5 comes with a library of two thousand graphics to illustrate common words and phrases.
- It also accepts picture files.
- Pictures appear as the user types or drags pictures into cells from the Picture Palette.
- Many grids are available online to work on different aspects of literacy.
- Windows and Mac
- $199.00

Greeting Card Software

- Greeting Card Software is readily available on CDs or thru online software sites.
- Clients create customized cards while practicing communication and cognitive skills.
- It's an ideal way to encourage social interaction and to foster relationships.
- Cards can be printed on paper or sent electronically.
- A review of this mainstream software can be found at http://greeting-card-software-review.toptenreviews.com/.
- There are several quality online greeting card sites:
    - www.bluemountain.com- which offers talking e-cards

- www.123greetings.com
- www.americangreetings.com
- www.hallmark.com.

HyperStudio 4.5
by Sunburst Learning, www.sunburst.com

- HyperStudio 4.5 uses brainstorming tools, visual organizers, project planners, desktop publishing features, and multimedia presentation capabilities.
- There are authoring tools for CD-ROMs and Web site development.
- Windows and Mac
- $69.95

Kidspiration 2.1
by Inspiration, www.inspiration.com

- Kidspiration 2.1 includes a library of 1,200 symbols to convey ideas and relationships.
- The Symbol Maker tool makes it easy for users to draw personalized symbols to include in graphic organizers.
- By choosing the Listen Tool, the user can hear text read aloud.
- Voice can be recorded.
- Windows and Mac
- $69.00

IntelliPics Studio 3
by IntelliTools, www.intellitools.com

- IntelliPics Studio 3 is a multimedia software tool with a range of activities across grade levels and content areas.
- It can be used to draw or paint and create storybooks.
- Users can create presentations with animated graphics, sounds (including MP3s), digital photos, movies, and links to the Internet.
- There is an expandable graphics collection with over 1,500 images, over 100 movie clips, 16 frame animations, and 200 sounds.
- Images, video, and recorded sound can be imported.
- Internet links can be added.
- There is an integrated word prediction to help with writing.
- Windows and Mac

- $139.95

KidPix Deluxe 4
by Riverdeep, www.broderbund.com

- KidPix Deluxe 4 is multimedia software that incorporates photos, text, sounds, and many special effects to design creative products.

- It begins with a blank screen with pull-down menus at the top of the screen and fourteen drawing tools on the left.

- Each tool has a corresponding sound, and the program has a feature that allows for the creation of additional sounds, so that users can input cues or instructions.

- The program's tools include over one hundred colored stamps of pictures; sound effects that can be turned off and on; an Electric Mixer that scrambles and animates images; a Wacky Brush that produces squiggles, dribbles, and other design elements; a random Paint Mixer that creates colorful patterns; and a Small Kids Mode for younger users.

- This program can be run in English or Spanish.

- Photos and graphics can be added.

- Windows or Mac

- $89.95 for the school edition and $34.99 for the home version

Photo Story 3
by Microsoft Corporation , www.microsoft.com

- This software can be used to create slideshows using digital photos. With a single click, the user can touch-up, crop, or rotate pictures. Add special effects, soundtracks, and voice narration to photo stories. Then, personalize them with titles and captions.

- Windows

- Free download

Pixie
by Tech4Learning, www.tech4learning.com

- Pixie is a creativity software with an array of paint and image editing tools.

- Voices can be recorded for narration and storytelling.

- Pictures can be exported to use in word processing and multimedia projects.

- Dozens of curriculum activities are included.

- Windows and Mac

- $44.95 for a single computer

PowerPoint 2003 and PowerPoint 2007
by Microsoft Corporation , www.microsoft.com

- PowerPoint is often purchased as part of the Microsoft Office Suite.
- It is most often used to produce presentations for meetings, but can effectively be used as an educational and therapy tool.
- It is possible to add voice, pictures, movies, custom animation, and sounds to produce talking books, slide show lessons and therapy activities.
- Windows and Mac
- $219.99

WebBlender
by Tech4Learning at www.tech4learning.com

- This software enables users to create Web sites with intuitive tools and an easy interface.
- Designs, images, links, buttons and text can be added without special coding.
- The user can import sounds, record voice or use text to speech.
- Windows and Mac
- $44.95

Sources for Pictures

There are many sources for pictures. Some software is available for purchase, while other pictures are available online for free. These pictures can be saved on a computer in Microsoft Word in the Clip Art Directory for easy access.

Software programs for purchase:

Title	Web Site	Price	PC	Mac
Boardmaker v 6	www.mayer-johnson.com	$299.00	x	
Boardmaker for Mac	www.mayer-johnson.com	$299.00		x
Boardmaker at Home	www.mayer-johnson.com	$149.00	x	
Eye-cons	http://kidaccess.com	$89.00	x	x
PCS Metafiles Deluxe	www.mayer-johnson.com	$199.00	x	x

Title	Web Site	Price	PC	Mac
Picture It v4.2	www.slatersoftware.com	$295.00	x	x
Picture This... Series	www.silverliningmm.com	$89.95	x	x
Places You Go, Things You Do	www.silverliningmm.com	$39.95	x	x

Boardmaker Version 6 and Boardmaker for Mac
by Mayer-Johnson, www.mayer-johnson.com

- Boardmaker is a communication and learning tool that contains over three thousand Picture Communication Symbols (PCSs) and over three hundred templates for creating schedules, devices, calendars, worksheets, and custom-made games and activities.

- Digital photos and drawings can be imported.

- Symbols and pictures can be resized and formatted for customization.

- Each symbol may be found and printed in multiple languages and can be copied with or without text.

- There are many products on the market to supplement this product.

- It can be used with 42 languages.

- Windows and Mac

- $299.00

Boardmaker at Home
by Mayer-Johnson, www.mayer-johnson.com

- Licensed for home use only.

- Offers less than the professional Boardmaker software, but does include more than 3,800 PCS in both color and black-and-white, all supported by 42 languages.

- Intended for use by families.

- Windows

- $149.00

Eye-cons
by KidAccess, http://kidaccess.com

- This CD includes full-color realistic images that are more abstract than photos and more concrete than those of Mayer-Johnson's Boardmaker or PCS.

- It includes more than one thousand images specifically designed for preschool-age and elementary school-aged children.

- Two-inch versions of each eye-con (no words, no grid) in two industry-standard formats (GIF and BMP) can be imported into Boardmaker or most other off-the-shelf word processing or graphics programs.

- Windows or Mac

- $89.00

PCS Metafiles Deluxe
by Mayer-Johnson, www.mayer-johnson.com

- This is a set of over seven thousand vector-drawn PCSs for use with Windows-compatible machines.

- Each picture is a separate file with its own file name and may be imported into other programs such as Clicker, PageMaker, and Corel Draw.

- The pictures in the PCS Metafiles come in black-and-white and color and are the same as the pictures in Boardmaker, plus all of the Addendum Libraries.

- Windows or Mac

- $199.00

Picture It v4.2
by Slater Software, www.slatersoftware.com

- Picture It is an easy-to-use program for adding pictures to text.

- It includes over six thousand Literacy Support Symbols with both black and white and color versions.

- There are built-in formatting options for making adapted books, worksheets, communication boards, and flashcards.

- It can be used in English or Spanish.

- It can be used with PixWriter to create a picture-based word processor.

- Windows or Mac

- $295.00

Picture This... Series
by Silver Lining Multimedia, www.silverliningmm.com

- Picture This... Pro contains over five thousand photos and a formatting program.

- It enables the user to search by initial, medial, and final sounds for easy creation of articulation cards.

- There are eight categories: chores, health, math, money, school, time, "What's different?" and "What's wrong?"

- Lotto boards with different-colored borders can be created using pictures, words, or sentences.

- Flash cards can be used for picture schedules, communication boards, and matching activities.

- This program can:
  - Search phonetically or by word
  - Print labels in English, French, German, Spanish, or Italian
  - Easily move and copy pictures
  - Print any custom-sized card with or without colored borders
  - Print colored labels above or below the picture

- Windows or Mac.

- $89.95.

Places You Go, Things You Do
by Silver Lining Multimedia, www.silverliningmm.com

- This software contains over 3,500 full-color photographs of everyday activities and places in the community.

- Like the photos from Picture This, many of those on this CD are shown against a plain white background.

- The photos on the CD are divided into fifty-eight folders within the following main topic areas: appointments, classes, dining, leisure, places, shopping, sports, and travel.

- Windows or Mac

- $39.95

Free Online Resources for Graphics

Clipart Directories

- http://freedigitalphotos.net/

- www.picsearch.com

- www.iconarchive.com

- www.iconbazaar.com

- www.kidsturncentral.com/clipart.htm

- www.free-clipart-pictures.net

- Image Tab on Search Engines such as Google.com, Dogpile.com, and Yahoo.com can be used as a free source of pictures. Unfortunately, when searching for pictures, these sites now display too many irrelevant and inappropriate images.

Imagine Symbols

available at www.imaginesymbols.com

- There are realistic symbols that are organized by core vocabulary words and 4,000 words grouped by category.

- Imagine Symbols are available for free as a download for non-commercial use. In order to download the symbols, the user needs to fill out a registration form.

- Free

Pics4Learning.com

by Tech4Learning.com, www.pics4learning.com

- This free online image collection includes over 20,000 pictures with no copyrights.

- It also features multi-level lesson plans written in conjunction with thematic digital images.

PictureSET Database

by SET-BC, www.setbc.org/pictureset/Default.aspx

- PictureSET is a collection of downloadable visual supports that can be used for both receptive and expressive communication.

- The collection is growing; it includes over one thousand files. PictureSET topic areas include community, health, holidays, home, mall, and school activities.

- This searchable database allows you to find a wide range of useful visual supports for different curriculum areas, activities, and events.

- SET-BC is a B.C. Ministry of Education Provincial Resource Program. It was established to assist school districts in educating students whose access to the curriculum is restricted primarily because of autism, physical disability, or visual impairment.

- Free

Speech Teach UK Clipart
http://www.speechteach.co.uk/p_resource/clipart/clipart_intro.htm

- This is a large selection of downloadable pictures which were either designed by a speech-language pathologist or found on the Internet.

- Words are grouped into categories such as initial sounds and topics such as clothing, animals and foods.

- Images printed directly from the browser will be quite small. To get a larger image right click picture and save image then import the image into your word processing package and then enlarge the image.

- Free

Tech/Syms
by Advanced Multimedia Devices, www.amdi.net/techsyms.htm

- Tech/Syms is a collection of pictorial symbols used for communication. It is based as WMF files for use with Advanced Multimedia Devices Tech/Overlay Designer software and other communication software applications.

- Each series features different categorical symbols such as foods, places, time and feelings.

- Free

Chapter 17:
Games and Free, Online, Interactive Activities

Many people believe that playing games is a waste of time. This could not be further from the truth. Traditional and computer-based games are often treatment material goldmines! Games can be used effectively during almost every treatment session and incorporated into independent practice programs.

There are many online sites as well as CDs which provide enjoyable interactive activities and games for practicing skills to reach treatment goals. It is often hard to distinguish between interactive multimedia sites designed for therapy and education and games for leisure and recreation. Board games, card games, strategy games, word games and even games of luck, when used appropriately, offer enormous benefits. Children may be more easily engaged in therapy and practice new skills without realizing that there is an educational process taking place. Adults can reduce stress, enjoy acquiring new skills, and find new ways to interact with others.

The following communication and cognitive treatment goal areas can be addressed during treatment with games and online interactive activities:

- Attention
- Concentration
- Direct Computer Access/Mouse manipulation
- Memory
- Problem solving
- Stress reduction
- Turn-taking
- Visual scanning

- Categorization
- Concept formation
- Initiation
- Planning and organization
- Sequencing
- Time management
- Verbal expression
- Word finding

New brain research shows that brain pathways improve with practice. It's helpful if we can find ways for clients to practice the skills they are working on in treatment with enjoyable activities. Games can be effective tools for both higher-level and lower-level clients. They need to be changed and adapted to meet the needs of the client. This can be accomplished by exploring and selecting options that are provided with the game, changing what the client is expected to do or by varying the amount of assistance provided during the game.

As with other treatment materials, keep in mind

- the goals of therapy,
- visual impairments,
- fine motor abilities,
- cognitive and communication strengths and weaknesses, and
- interests of the client.

Traditional Games

Listed below are traditional games that lend themselves to effective use in treatment. It's beyond the scope of this guide to describe each game and review potential accommodations and adaptations for particular types of clients and goals. Most of these items can be found online through search engines or at local toy stores. Rules need to be adapted and created, and activities modified, to make them appropriate for each person. Adding an expressive component to describe actions, such as having the client name a color or number, or describe what they are doing, or why one is an example of tailoring the activity to help reach a goal.

Many types of traditional games can be helpful for therapy. Many of them now have computer equivalents. This listing is provided to heighten your awareness of the many available treatment materials many of us already may have at our disposal.

Board Games

- Backgammon
- Clue
- Lotto
- Trivial Pursuit

- Blokus
- Four in a Row
- Parcheesi

- Checkers
- Guess Who
- Sequence

Card Games

- Bingo
- Crazy Eights
- Poker

- Blackjack
- Go Fish
- Solitaire

- Concentration
- Rummy
- Uno

Guessing Games

- Battleship
- Hangman
- Name that Tune
- Charades
- I spy
- Pictionary
- Guess Who
- Mastermind
- Twenty Questions

Word Games and Puzzles

- Anagrams
- Categories
- Hangman
- Scategories
- Upwords
- Apples to Apples
- Charades
- Jigsaw Puzzles
- Scrabble
- Word Search
- Boggle
- Crosswords
- Malarky
- Taboo

Resources for Adapted Games

Some clients may benefit from certain products that were created to make games easier to play for people with disabilities. Products may be made larger and easier to manipulate. There are also games that were produced to be used to improve communication and cognition. Please refer to the following listings for more information:

- **Dynamic Living**, www.dynamic-living.com (search under games)
- **KY Enterprises**, www.quadcontrol.com- Adaptive Products for Independent Living and Recreation
- **Assistive Technology Partners**, http://www.uchsc.edu/atp/adapted_home/play.htm#comp
- **Audiogames.net**, www.audiogames.net- Games for the visually impaired.

New Educational Gaming Technologies

We typically think of desktop and laptop computers and the Internet when contemplating which games to use in treatment. Recent technological developments have broadened the possibilities. Gameboys, XBox, Nintendo, Smart phones, Pocket PCs, Palms, and other devices for playing games have become commonplace—for both children and adults. A few of them lend themselves particularly well to helping people who have communication and cognitive challenges.

Big Brain Academy
by Nintendo at www.bigbrainacademy.com

- The Nintendo DS handheld game system is used to play Big Brain Academy. It is available wherever video games and most home entertainment products are sold. Examples include Toys R Us, Best Buy, and Target.

- New users first take a five-category quiz and test their brain's ability to think, memorize, compute, analyze and identify.

- This game features 15 activities that test brain powers in areas like logic, memory, math and analysis. Up to eight people can play with a single game card, and each activity takes less than a minute to complete.

- Nintendo DS

- $19.99

Brain Age
by Nintendo at www.brainage.com

- Brain Age is played with the Nintendo DS rotated 90 degrees to the right so the system more closely resembles a book.

- Input comes via the touch screen, stylus, and occasionally the microphone.

- Progress is tracked.

- Brain Age features activities designed to help stimulate the brain with a wide variety of activities such as solving simple math problems, counting people going in and out of a house simultaneously, drawing pictures on the Nintendo DS touch screen, and reading classic literature out loud.

- $19.99 at stores such as Best Buy or Target.

LeapFrog
available at www.leapfrog.com

- LeapFrog produces a large number of educational products which can be very effective in treatment.

- There are preschool products such as My First LeapPad, Grade school products such as the Leapster and LeapPad Learning System and products for older students such as the Fly Pen and iQuest.

Gaming Software

There is a wide variety of gaming software. As with other types of technology, gaming technology is advancing rapidly. With a creative clinician, many of the new products can be used to help people improve their communication and cognition. Some are more educational in nature than others. All can creatively be used to improve communication and cognition. Here is a brief listing of the many mainstream games that can be integrated into treatment:

- Battleship by Hasbro Interactive
- Boggle by Hasbro Interactive
- Hoyle Board and Card Games
- I Spy Series by Scholastic
- Jumpstart Series by Vivendi Universal
- Oregon Trail by Encore Software
- Reader Rabbit Series by The Learning Company
- Scrabble by Hasbro Interactive
- Sims by Electronic Arts
- Wheel of Fortune by Atari
- Yahtzee by Hasbro Interactive

Many games can be used in different ways to work on different goal areas. These sites may be helpful when searching for games:

- www.Amazon.com
- www.bestbuy.com
- www.educational-software-directory.net/games
- www.childrenssoftwareonline.com
- http://boardgamecentral.com
- www.knowledgeadventure.com
- www.smartkidssoftware.com

Especially appropriate for children are two mainstream pediatric educational software titles:

JumpStart Software
by Knowledge Adventure, http://www.knowledgeadventure.com

- The JumpStart adventures revolve around kid-friendly themes.
- Players may take an assessment test prior to beginning play to determine appropriate levels of difficulty for a variety of skills and automatically adjust to the child's pace. Most activities offer several levels of play.
- Enjoyable activities build skills in math, science, reading, and art.
- There are grade and subject titles for ages 6 months to 12 years.

Humongous Entertainment Software
available at http://www.humongous.com

- Humongous Entertainment produces quite a few kid-friendly problem solving programs.

- Examples include: Pajama Sam, Freddie Fish, Backyard Football and Putt-Putt.

- The programs require the children to accumulate specific items, navigate a number of locations, play games and use their memory and reasoning skills to help the on-screen characters achieve goals.

Games Already Installed on Windows

Windows XP and Windows Vista come with games installed. To find them, click Start, choose All Programs, and select Games. Some require an Internet connection. For details regarding XP games go to www.microsoft.com/windowsxp/using/games/getstarted/inboxgames.mspx.

- FreeCell
- Minesweeper
- Solitaire
- Hearts
- Spider Solitaire
- Pinball

Spider Solitaire (the easiest level) and Solitaire (made easier with turning over 1 page at a time and showing the Outline Dragging options) are very helpful when helping clients become more adept at using the mouse, to improve visual-perceptual skills, and to practice verbal skills.

Windows Vista includes updates of the classic Windows games, plus several new ones including Chess Titans, InkBall, Mahjong Titans, and Purple Place.

For details regarding Vista games, go to http://www.microsoft.com/windows/products/windowsvista/features/games.mspx to learn more.

Online, Free, Interactive Programs

The following free online resources do not require membership or fees. Some require logins and passwords. They may require Macromedia Shockwave or a Java platform — both of which can be downloaded at no charge. Depending on the Internet connection speed, most downloads are fast. Some games are played alone, while others engage the play of others who are online. Clinicians can adapt them all to work toward therapy goals. Spend a bit of time checking out the sites to determine which are best for your client and how they should be used. They can provide hundreds of hours of practice working on communication and cognition.

Web Sites With Directories and Extensive Databases of Free, Online, Interactive Programs

Net Connection for Communication Disorders and Sciences
available at http://www.mnsu.edu/comdis/kuster2/sptherapy.html

- This is a comprehensive Internet Guide which offers an extensive database for Web sites for online activities and information.

Awesomlibrary.org
available at www.awesomelibrary.org/Office/Main/New_and_Exciting/Games/Word_Games.html

- This Directory of Games provides an extensive database of resources that have been reviewed and found to be of high quality.

Berit's Best Sites for Children
available at www.beritsbest.com

- This site reviews and provides links to over one thousand sites with materials and activities for children.
- It also provides a rating for each site, as well as some online activities including interactive stories, coloring books, and funny sounds.

Call Centre
available at http://callcentre.education.ed.ac.uk/index.html

- The Call Centre offers jokes for communication, for people who use voice output communication aids.

Cbeebies
available at www.bbc.co.uk/cbeebies

- CBeebies online has many pre-school characters and lots of fun games, stories and activities.

Children's Storybooks Online
available at http://www.magickeys.com/books

- Free online talking e-books are provided with pictures categorized for young children, older children and young adults.
- This site also offers online jigsaw puzzles, riddles, and online games.

ESL Independent Study Lab
available at www.lclark.edu/~krauss/toppicks/toppicks.html

- This site contains over 250 Internet resources categorized by skill area and language level for English literacy learning.

Gameaquarium
available at www.gamequarium.com

- This site offers over 1,500 links to online games that are categorized by core content.

- Kids can practice skills with scores and times to record on learning logs.

- Language arts activities include word fun, vocabulary games, parts of speech, sentence structure, spelling, and punctuation.

Hiyah.net
available at www hiyah.net

- This Web site offers free software for children who need cause-effect programs.

- The programs are based on high interest subjects, such as nursery rhymes, holidays, and birthday themes.

- The programs can operate on their own by pressing the spacebar.

Oxford University Press
available at www.oup.com/elt/students/?cc=gb

- Oxford University Press offers a large number of Web sites with interactive language-learning games for all ages.

TopEnglishTeaching.com
available at www.topenglishteaching.com

- This site is a search engine for teachers of English.

- The user inputs the level, age, skill, and topic for treatment, the site presents helpful Web sites.

- These Web sites include games, activities, worksheets, songs, lesson plans, readings, and listening activities.

Yahooligans
available at http://kids.yahoo.com/games/index

- This site provides direct links to a wide variety of word related games.

- It has screened the many online games for sites that are appropriate for children.

- They include anagrams, crossword puzzles, hangman, mad Libs, and word searches.

Free Interactive Web Sites

Below is a brief description of sites that are appropriate for working with clients to improve communication and cognitive skills.

www.1-language.com

- This is a comprehensive ESL site that offers free games, including a memory and matching game.
- In it, the client selects a topic such as body parts. He or she then selects a block, and the squares are turned over and the picture is named.

www.allgamesfree.com

- This site offers a wide variety of free arcade games, card games, puzzle and word games, sports games, and interactive trivia games.
- Once a client has registered, he or she will be able to create a custom "My Games" page with favorite games.

www.aarp.org/games

- AARP Online Games and Puzzles feature online puzzles, jigsaws, and other interactive games.
- There are clear instructions with minimal advertising interruptions.

www.allinplay.com

- A few multi-player games are fully accessible and were designed to work with a screen reader or screen magnifier.
- There is a free trial period, and then access to popular card games cost less than $8.00 a month.
- The player can practice against the computer or play against others on Windows PCs.

www.arcess.com

- These simple switch games are easy to play and are designed to be widely accessible for players who have muscular dystrophy, cerebral palsy, spinal injury, head injury, or other physical disabilities.
- They can be played as single switch games, speech recognition games, and expanded keyboard games.

www.askforkids.com

- This site provides educational fun and games, news resources for kids, and books to click on for study help in academic areas.

www.bry-backmanor.org

- This site contains a vast collection of games for download on a Mac and materials to use with children who have special needs.

www.coolmath.com

- This site contains many math and cognitive games.

www.dotolearn.com

- Do2Learn offers ready-to-use communication tools, games, and drawing activities for children with special needs.

www.englishclub.com

- In this ESL clubhouse produced in England, there is a section for games.
- Words are grouped by categories, such as animals, business, and sports.
- They include crosswords, jumbled words, matching games, and a typing test.

http://a4esl.org

- This site features quizzes, tests, exercises, and puzzles to help learn English.
- Specific lessons offer grammar and vocabulary quizzes, and crossword puzzles.

www.englishforum.com/00/interactive

- This site offers a wide selection for grammar, vocabulary and idioms practice.

www.funbrain.com

- This site has math, spelling, and creative writing games.
- Each section allows users to start the game over, to switch levels, or to return to the home page to select another game.

www.gotofreegames.com

- This site offers puzzles, card games, and other language and cognitive based interactive games.

www.uiowa.edu/%7Eacadtech/phonetics/#

- This site shows diagrams with movement and sound to assist with teaching manner and place of producing sounds.

www.jigzone.com

- This is a great site for puzzles with a wide variety of levels.
- You can determine the pictures, number of pieces, and shape.

www.juniorsweb.com

- There are many ready-to-go communication treatment activities that focus on articulation, language, and emergent literacy.

www.languagegames.org

- After selecting a language and topic, there are crosswords, hangman, and word search games to play.

www.learningplanet.com

- LearningPlanet.com provides a wide variety of fun learning activities, educational games, printable worksheets, and powerful tools.

- Educational games are provided for kids from pre-kindergarten to sixth grade.

- Users can choose a grade level and get a list of games designed to improve their learning skills and proficiency in many different subjects.

http://literactive.com

- Literactive offers free online reading material for pre-school, kindergarten and Grade 1 students.

- The program is comprised of carefully leveled animated guided readers, comprehensive phonic activities and supplemental reading material.

- A complete phonemic and syllabic breakdown of every word in the stories is provided enabling each child to decode the written text working alone or in small classroom groups.

- ESL versions for the reading material are available for download.

- Starting with initial nursery rhymes, it moves through pre-reading activities, alphabet awareness, letter sounds, short vowels, CVC word blending, initial blends, long vowels and all the phonic activities critical for developing early reading skills.

- All the material is available for free from this site, but registration is required.

www.manythings.org

- This site includes quizzes, word games, word puzzles, proverbs, slang expressions, anagrams, a random-sentence generator, and other computer-assisted, language-learning activities.

www.mcps.k12.md.us/curriculum/pep/teachercreate.html

- This site includes communication boards and worksheets, adapted books and songs, IntelliPics games, IntelliTalk II activities, and many additional resources.

www.msngames.com

- This site offers a wide selection of board and card games that are especially easy to access and learn.

- It also provides hints, good game descriptions, and easy browsing.

www.parentpals.com/gossamer/pages/Special_Education_Games/index.html

- Parentpals offers a wide variety of Internet educational and therapy games to enhance learning and language skills which are organized in levels of difficulty.

www.pbskids.org

- This site features many games and learning activities related to PBS shows such as Arthur, Barney, and Dragon Tales.

www.pogo.com

- Pogo offers a wide variety of games and helpful directions. There are loads of free games of all different types: cards, puzzles, word, casino, arcade, and sports.

www.primarygames.com

- This site offers interactive online games for elementary-age children.

- It is very colorful, requires a Java-enabled browser, and has commercial banner ads.

- The site covers language arts, math, science, and social studies skills.

www.quia.com

- The Quintessential Instructional Archive (QUIA) provides templates for creating many different types of online games.

- Activities include: flashcards, matching, concentration (memory), word search, hangman, challenge board, and rags to riches (a quiz-show style trivia game) as well as tools for creating online quizzes.

- There are free worksheets, online games, and downloadable games.

www.readwritething.org

- ReadWriteThink is a partnership between the International Reading Association (IRA), the National Council of Teachers of English (NCTE), and the Verizon Foundation.

- This site offers teaching lessons, Web resources, and student materials.

www.sadlier-oxford.com/phonics/control_page/front2.htm

- This site offers a wide variety of games grouped by grade level and type of task.
- There are games related to phonics, antonyms, synonyms, analogies, and word study skills.

www.scholastic.com

- This site offers games and activities for kids; activities, information, and advice for parents; lessons, activities, and tools for teachers; and trends, products, and solutions for administrators.
- There are many free online reading and writing projects.

http://school.discovery.com/brainboosters

- School Discovery offers a categorized archive of challenging Brain Boosters.
- It has activities work to improve categorizations, lateral thinking, logic, number and math play, reasoning, spatial awareness, and word and letter play.

www.starfall.com

- This is an elementary-level site for phonetic spelling and learning to read.
- There are over twenty free interactive stories with a variety of tasks for the emergent reader.
- It is phonics based and requires the child to be able to click and drag.

http://teacher.scholastic.com/clifford1

- Scholastic provides stories about Clifford that include buttons to have lines of text read and the ability to select words to add to the story.

www.thepuzzleplayer.com

- This site offers free daily puzzles.

www.tumblebooks.com

- The Tumblebook library includes an online collection of animated talking-picture books, reading comprehension quizzes, educational games, and professional resources.

www.vocabulary.com

- This site has interactive vocabulary puzzles and activities that use Latin and Greek "roots and cells" to help decode words.

- They are separated into three levels of difficulty.

- Seven links to current exercises include Fill in the Blanks, Definition Match, Synonym and Antonym Encounters, Crosswords, Word Finds, True/False, and Word Stories.

http://vocabulary.co.il

- This site offers easy to use crosswords, word search, hangman, Jumble, and a matching game.

- Each activity has three levels of difficulty and provides a wide variety of topics.

Chapter 18:
Internet Communication Tools

The Web is full of valuable information. The Internet is changing the way that we find and present information. As professionals, we must learn to use these new tools and integrate them into our treatment practices as well as our daily lives. Many of our younger clients are already using podcasts, instant messaging, text messages, and social networking sites. In order to help people of all ages with communication and cognitive deficits, we need to understand these communication methods to help our clients benefit from them along with the rest of society. We must take advantage of blogs, podcasts, listservs, and text messaging to improve our client's rehabilitation and education. In this chapter, examples of communication tools are highlighted that can be helpful for professional development and when planning and providing treatment.

Here is a list of these communication tools:

- Announcement lists
- Chat rooms

- E-learning and distance education
- Games
- Instant messaging
- RSS feeds
- Text messages
- Videoweb
- Wikis

- Blogs: Web logs
- Discussion groups, listservs, newsgroups, and bulletin boards
- E-mail
- Immersive environments
- Podcasts
- Social networking sites
- Video conferencing
- Web sites

Announcement Lists

- Announcement lists, also known as one-way distribution lists, are computer lists that send subscribers information, but do not have members interact with other list members.

- There is automatic distribution to registered participants.

- There are many lists available for education and rehabilitation professionals. Lists may be found by referring to the many Web sites for organizations and associations referred to in Chapter 19.

Blogs: Web Logs

- A blog is a Web page made up of short, frequently updated postings that are arranged chronologically.

- Blog posts are like instant messages to the Web. Blog users can post, modify, or delete their own posts to the blog Web site. A blog may be set up so that users can comment on posts made by other members.

- Blogs are a great way to keep up with the latest technological advances. Brian Friedlander writes an informative blog about assistive technology at http://assistivetek.blogspot.com/.

Chat rooms

- A chat room is an online site in which people can talk by posting messages to people who are on the same site at the same time.

- Sometimes the messages are moderated.

- There are different rooms for people who have different interests.

- A very active chat room for stroke survivors can be found at www.strokechat.net.

- A chat room for youth and young adults with learning disabilities can be found at http://www.ldpride.net/chatguidelines.htm.

Discussion Groups, Listservs, Electronic Mailing Lists, and Bulletin Boards

- Discussion groups or lists allow for ongoing discussions among members, who are not online at the same time. They facilitate interaction among members because they enable members to post questions, comments, suggestions or answers to a large number of people without everyone being available at the same time.

- Some are moderated while others automatically accept all postings.

- They are typically fully or partially automated through the use of special mailing list software. Some mailing lists archive their postings and these archives are available on the Internet for browsing.

- Some mailing lists are open to anyone who wants to join them, while others require an approval from the list owner in order for someone to join. Some are free; others require a fee.

A few examples include:

- AAPPSPA — The American Academy of Private Practice in Speech Pathology and Audiology at www.aappspa.org. This listserv requires membership.

- Special Interest Divisions (SIDS) thru the American Speech and Hearing Association (www.asha.org) which also require membership.

- QIAT (Quality Indicators for Assistive Technology) at http://sweb.uky.edu/~jszaba0/QIAT.html.

E-Learning and Distance Education (Internet/Web-Based Training)

- Distance Education is designed to be used remotely over the Internet.

- Teachers and students may communicate either at times of their own choosing and proceed at their own pace by using printed and electronic media, or use technology that permits communication in real time.

- Professionals can obtain continuing education in their home or at work without the travel costs and inconveniences.

- These sites are becoming increasingly popular. In Chapter 19, "Online Support, Information, and Discussion Groups," sites are listed that offer assistive technology training programs. Many are online.

More information about some of the online training and distance education opportunities can be found at:

- The National Assistive Technology Technical Assistance Partnership (NATTAP) at http://www.resna.org/taproject/library/pubs/DistEdResGuide.htm.

- OnlineCeus.com at www.onlineceus.com

- SpeechPathology.com at www.speechpathology.com

- EASI –(Equal Access to Software and Information), www.easi.cc/workshop.htm

- ATTO (The Assistive Technology Training Online) Project at the University of Buffalo at http://atto.buffalo.edu

E-mail

- Users can type and send written messages over the Internet to another person or group of people by use of e-mail addresses.

- The recipient of the message can read the message at a convenient time using a computer or handheld communication device.

- Chapter 15 "Adapted E-mail, Search Engines and Web Browsers" reviews specific ways that e-mail can be used with people who have communication and cognitive deficits.

- Popular e-mail hosts include AOL (www.aol.com), Yahoo! (www.yahoo.com), Comcast (www.comcast.com), and Gmail (www.gmail.com.).

Games

- There are many games available online designed specifically for education and personal motivation.

- Refer to Chapter 17, "Games and Free Online Interactive Activities."

Immersive Environments

- These Web sites with virtual environments and avatars (online virtual bodies) where participants engage each other through the persona of the figure representing them are growing in popularity.

- An example is Second Life, http://secondlife.com/. Second Life is a 3-D virtual world entirely built and owned by its residents.

- Since opening to the public in 2003, it has grown and today is inhabited by nearly 200,000 people from around the globe. There are shopping malls, events, homes, lands of different types, and participants contribute content, buildings, and other digital creations.

Instant Messaging

- Instant Messaging is a method of Internet and phone communication that allows two or more people to "chat" by sending messages back and forth immediately.

- Instant Messaging users set up "buddy lists" and see when their family, friends, and associates are online and available to exchange messages.

- Sending a message opens up a small window where the sender and recipient both can see the messages being sent.

- AIM (AOL Instant Messenger) is a popular free instant messaging service. It can be downloaded for free at www.aim.com.

Podcasts

- A podcast is like an Internet radio show that you can download and listen to at your convenience or listen to directly from the Web site.

- The majority of podcasts are MP3 files, which means that a person can listen to them on any MP3 player or on a computer.

- As the use of iPods and other handheld listening devices becomes more prevalent in our society, this new technology is becoming more commonplace.

- You can download one of any number of free software programs to your computer such as iTunes. The programs can be programmed to capture particular podcasts.

- Depending on the configuration, when the program finds a new episode of one of your podcasts, it will either automatically download the show to your computer, or just capture a brief description of the episode, so you can decide whether you want to download it or not.

To give you a feel for what podcasts are like, check out these links:

- The podcast for Parents by Parents of Kids with Learning Disabilities, www.ldpodcast.com.

- The voice of parents of children with autism spectrum disorders, www.autismvoice.com

- Health and medicine podcast from John's Hopkins Medicine, http://www.hopkinsmedicine.org/mediall/Podcasts.html

- Education and Technology Today A Podcast Series, http://inst.cl.uh.edu/PodCasts/index.asp

- Disability 411, http://disability411.jinkle.com/podcastq.htm

- ADD Resources, www.addresources.org/adhd_webcasts.php

RSS Feeds

- Feeds help connect Web authors and their audience.

- Authors can choose to notify others automatically of new entries or changes to part of a Web site or blog by creating a "feed."

- Others may choose to be notified automatically of those new entries or changes by subscribing to "feeds."

- Choosing to receive notification is called "subscribing" to the feed for that part of that Web site. Along with notification, the subscriber usually gets some form of direct access to the new or changed material.

- New browsers have built-in feed detection, subscription and management.

- An example can be found at CNN.com which will send out headline news.

Social Networking Sites

- Social networking sites allow people to create profiles about themselves and connect or network with other people's profiles.

- Once they have networked with a friend they can then view the profiles of their friend's friends. As they connect with more and more people their social network expands.

- These networks can then be used for fun, for connecting specific groups, for arranging activities, and for networking.

- Some popular social networking sites include MySpace.com, Facebook.com, and LinkedIn.com.

Text Messaging

- Text messaging is a communication mode that allows users to exchange messages up to 160 characters.

- The short messages are sent to a smart phone, pager, PDA, or other handheld device.

- There is a new written language to minimize keystrokes that has become popular with the rise of instant messaging, chat rooms, and text messaging. To learn this new lingo go, to webopedia.com/quick_ref/textmessageabbreviations.asp.

- It is especially helpful when talking on the phone is inappropriate or inconvenient and e-mailing is not available.

- Young people often now would rather send text messages, post messages on social sites, and send instant messages than call someone on the phone or send an e-mail to communicate.

Video Conferencing

- A videoconference is a set of interactive telecommunication technologies that allows two or more locations to interact via two-way video and audio transmissions at the same time.

- It promotes learning by providing a 2-way communication platform and providing access to specialists to people in remote or isolated places.

- One example is Skype at www.skype.com.

Video on the Web

- This technology enables users to view videos over the Internet

- The Google Video Store is a video distribution service that offers paid content alongside free videos, and lets users upload their own video clips and charge for them.

- Streaming media is a technology that delivers audio, video, images, and text to the user without downloading the entire file at one time. It feeds the user only the portion of the file they need at the moment, and does not save the entire file to the user's computer.

- YouTube offers users the opportunity at no cost to broadcast videos on the Internet. The video can be uploaded, tagged and shared. It can also be used to view thousands of original videos which were uploaded by community members. There are many video groups to connect with people of similar interests. More information can be found at www.youtube.com.

Video Podcasts

- Video podcasts are becoming more common.

- Users can subscribe to these, but in order to play them, they need to use a computer or have a player that can show video, such as the video iPod.

- For a great example check out The University of Wisconsin-Madison Campus Division of Information Technology videopodcast at http://www.doit.wisc.edu/accessibility/video/.

Web Sites

- A Web site is a collection of Web pages all connected to the same home page.

- A Web page is a screen full of information. Web sites together are referred to as the "World Wide Web" (www).

- The pages of a Web site start from the homepage. There can be links provided to allow the user to move from one page to another.

- Some Web sites require a subscription to some or all of the contents while others offer open access. Some subscriptions are free and some require a fee.

Web Site Accessibility

- Web site accessibility is becoming more important as Internet access becomes mainstream and more people with disabilities are learning to use assistive technology to obtain information and interact with online society.

- In the US, it is now the law that federally funded Web sites must be Section 508 Compliant, that is, accessible. More information on this law can be found at www.section508.gov.

- For more information about accessibility issues check out:
  - Web Accessibility Initiative, http://www.w3.org/WAI/
  - Dive Into Accessibility, http://diveintoaccessibility.org/
- There are companies for hire to assist with helping businesses make sure their Web sites comply with these regulations. One example is Accessible Computing at www.accessiblecomputing.com.

Wikis

- A Wiki is a collaborative Web site comprised of the collective work of many authors.
- It allows users to easily upload, edit, and interlink pages.
- A popular wiki is Wikipedia at www.wikipedia.com — an open content encyclopedia. It is offered in many languages.

Chapter 19:
Online Support, Information, and Discussion Groups

(Many of the sites in this chapter are posted online at www.ittsguides.com and www.innovativespeech.com for easy access. They will be updated regularly.)

In addition to the many ways that the Internet can be used to enhance direct treatment for communication and cognition, it is an affordable and efficient way to access support and information for our clients as well as for our own professional development. Unfortunately, many people are not aware that these helpful online resources exist.

As a word of caution, clients and professionals need keep a wary eye on what they learn online. While the Internet is a worthwhile and efficient source of information, it isn't well regulated. It's critical that everyone evaluate sites to determine if they are legitimate and trustworthy. Suggestions for evaluating Web sites can be found on the Schwab Foundation's site at the following Web site: www.schwablearning.org/articles.asp?r=429.

The Internet can be used to do the following tasks:

- Link people with online and local support groups.

- Access written literature regarding treatment approaches and research studies.

- Assist clinicians with appropriate referral sources and help clients find the help they need.

- Connect clients and clinicians with vendors who provide helpful products.

- Provide an ongoing source of professional development for clinicians and continued information about new treatment techniques and products for clients.

Because the Internet is constantly evolving, sites frequently appear and disappear. The Internet addresses provided here are current at the time of publication, but may change at any time. Many Web sites are listed in this chapter that can be helpful to professionals who assist people with communication and cognitive disorders. Many hours were spent researching and exploring these sites, but undoubtedly others may have been missed. These sites are numerous and are organized in this chapter into the following categories:

- Sites offering comprehensive information about multiple disability groups

- Sites with information grouped by diagnosis and disability

- Sites with information about products to promote independent living

- Sites offering technology training and information

- Sites grouped by profession

Sites Offering Comprehensive Information About Multiple Disability Groups

American Disability Association
available at www.ada.gov

- The ADA Home Page provides access to Americans with Disabilities Act (ADA) regulations, information, and suggestions.

Council for Exceptional Children (CEC)
available at www.cec.sped.org

- The largest international professional organization dedicated to improving the educational success of students with disabilities or gifts.

- CEC advocates for appropriate government policies, sets professional standards, provides continuous professional development, advocates for newly and historically underserved individuals with exceptionalities, and helps professionals obtain conditions and resources necessary for effective professional practice.

Disability 411
available at http://disability411.jinkle.com/podcastq.htm

- Disability 411 offers a podcast for disability professionals.

- It provides audio workshops, interviews and information on disability-related topics for those who work with individuals with disabilities.

- Information is also of interest for individuals with disabilities and their families.

- It is hosted by Beth Case, a disability counselor with 10 years of experience in postsecondary disability services.

DiscoverySchool.com
available at http://school.discovery.com/schrockguide/index.html

- Kathy Schrock's Guide for Educators is a categorized list of sites useful for enhancing curriculum and professional growth.

- It is updated often to include what she perceives to be the best sites for teaching and learning.

International Center for Disability Resources on the Internet
available at http://icdri.org

- ICDRI's mission is to collect a global knowledge base of quality disability resources and best practices and to provide education, outreach and training based on these core resources.

- The site can be translated automatically and is Web enabled.

Medline Plus
available at www.nlm.nih.gov/medlineplus

- MedlinePlus offers information and helps answer health questions by bringing together authoritative information from the National Library of Medicine (NLM), the National Institutes of Health (NIH), and other government agencies and health-related organizations.

Medscape
available at www.medscape.com

- Medscape's mission is to provide clinicians and other healthcare professionals with timely comprehensive and relevant clinical information to improve patient care.

Hardin Meta Directory of Internet Health Sources
available at www.lib.uiowa.edu/hardin/md/index.html

- This comprehensive site is maintained by the University of Iowa's Hardin Health Science Library.

- Information is arranged by subject clusters such as speech disorders, stroke, or autism.

- There is also an extensive database of related pictures.

- It provides links to associated Web sites of the chosen topic by showing what others in the subject often clicked.

HealingWell.com
available at www.healingwell.com

- HealingWell.com is a community and information resource for patients, caregivers, and families coping with diseases, disorders, and chronic illnesses.

- This site provides articles, news, information, video Web casts, message forums, chat rooms, e-mail, books, and a resource directory.

Health A to Z
available at www.healthatoz.com

- This is a consumer-oriented directory of rated sites in the area of health and medicine.

The Gerontological Society of America (GSA)
available at www.geron.org/online.html

- The GSA is a nonprofit professional organization with more than five thousand members in the field of aging.

- It provides researchers, educators, practitioners, and policy makers with opportunities to understand, advance, integrate, and use basic and applied research on aging to improve the quality of life as one ages.

- This site provides a comprehensive listing of helpful Web sites.

The Family Center on Technology and Disability
available at www.fctd.info

- The Family Center is a resource designed to support organizations and programs that work with families of children and youth with disabilities.

National Institute on Deafness and Other Communication Disorders (NIDCD)
available at www.nidcd.nih.gov

- This is the National Institutes of Health's division for research pertaining to hearing, balance, smell, taste, voice, speech, and language.

- Health information topics include a directory of related associations, helpful information, and resources.

Sites With Information Grouped by Diagnosis and Disability

(Technology Treatment Tips for clients grouped by diagnosis and area of disability were included in Chapter 3.)

AAC Users

- Augmentative Communication On-Line Users Group (ACOLUG) is a listserv created to exchange ideas, information and experiences on augmentative communication by people from all over the world.

- The listserv and its archives can be accessed from http://disabilities.temple.edu/programs/assistive/acolug.

Accent Reduction

(see also English Language Learners)

- American Accent Training, www.americanaccent.com
- Dave's ESL Café Web Guide, www.eslcafe.com
- International Phonetic Association, www.arts.gla.ac.uk/IPA/ipa.html
- The Speech Accent Archive, http://accent.gmu.edu

Alzheimer's Disease

(see also Brain Injury)

- Alzheimer's Association, www.alz.org
- National Institute on Aging Caregiver Guide,
  www.nia.nih.gov/Alzheimers/Publications/caregiverguide.htm
- Discussion Group:
  - Alzheimer forum for patients, professionals and family caregivers, researchers, public policymakers, students, and anyone with an interest in Alzheimer's or related dementia disorders in older adults. Subscribe to the list by sending e-mail to majordomo@wubios.wustl.edu with the message: subscribe alzheimer firstname lastname. To communicate with the list, send e-mail to alzheimer@wubios.wustl.edu.

Amyotrophic Lateral Sclerosis

(see also ALS or Lou Gehrig's Disease)

- The ALS Association, www.alsa.org
- Communication Independence for the Neurologically Impaired, www.cini.org
- Amyotrophic Lateral Sclerosis Resources, www.alslinks.com

Aneurysm

- The Brain Aneurysm Foundation, www.bafound.org

Aphasia

(see also Stroke)

- National Aphasia Association, www.aphasia.org
- Aphasia Now, www.aphasianow.org

- York-Durham Aphasia Centre, www.ydac.on.ca
- Talkback Association for Aphasia,
  http://www.aphasia.asn.au/aphasiafriendly/index.htm
- Discussion Group:
    - http://groups.yahoo.com/group/Aphasia/- The Aphasia mailing list was set up to share information, experiences, questions, knowledge, feelings, etc. etc. with respect to Aphasia.

Apraxia

- Childhood Apraxia of Speech Association, www.apraxia-kids.org
- Cherab Foundation, www.cherab.org / www.speechville.com
- Dyspraxia Association, www.dyspraxiafoundation.org.uk
- Discussion Groups:
    - http://health.groups.yahoo.com/group/phonologicaltherapy explores issues related to developmental phonological disorders, childhood apraxia of speech, and other childhood, speech sound disorders, and their clinical management.
    - http://health.groups.yahoo.com/group/phonologicaltherapy/- Members explore theoretical and research issues related to developmental phonological disorders, childhood apraxia of speech, and other childhood speech sound disorders, and their clinical management.

Asperger's Syndrome

- Online Asperger's Syndrome Information and Support,
  www.udel.edu/bkirby/asperger/

Attention Deficit Disorder (ADD)

- Children and Adults With Attention Deficit Disorder (CHADD), www.chadd.org
- Attention Deficit Disorder Resources, www.addresources.org
- Discussion Group
    - http://groups.yahoo.com/group/ADHD-ODD — This list is for parents of children who are, or who are suspected of being, ADD/ADHD with, or without ODD, as well as other disorders.

Autistic Spectrum Disorders

- Autism and PDD Support Network, www.autism-pdd.net

- Autism Society of America, www.autism-society.org

- Autism Speaks, www.autismspeaks.org

- Center for the Study of Autism, www.autism.org

- The Cody Center for Autism and Developmental Disabilities, www.codycenter.org

- Cure Autism Now, www.cureautismnow.org

- Discussion Groups:

  - ANI-L. Autism and autistic-like abnormalities are discussed at the Autism Network International's list. To subscribe, send the message: subscribe ani-l firstname lastname to listserv@listserv.syr.edu. To post your message to the entire list, send e-mail to ani-l@listserv.syr.edu.

  - Autism Educators, http://groups.yahoo.com/group/autismeducators/— This group is open to practitioners involved in the education of children with ASD who share two perspectives: firstly, that the world-view of people with autism is one that deserves to be respected and valued; and secondly, that no single teaching approach or technique is appropriate for teaching most or all children with ASD.

Blind

(see Low Vision)

Brain Injury

- Brain Injury Association of America, www.biausa.org

- Brain Injury Resource Center, www.headinjury.com

- Brain Injury Society, www.bisociety.org

- Traumatic Brain Injury Resources Guide, www.neuroskills.com

- Brain Fitness Channel, http://bfc.positscience.com

- Discussion Groups:

  - http://health.groups.yahoo.com/group/ABINews2U. This discussion group is designed to inform, educate, and enlighten others about TBI (Traumatic Brain Injury) or ABI (Acquired Brain Injury)

  - http://health.groups.yahoo.com/group/Traumatic_Brain_Injury/. This discussion group is dedicated to helping people learn about the major milestones on the road to recovery and providing assistance with resources.

Brain Tumor

- National Brain Tumor Foundation, www.braintumor.org

Central Auditory Processing Deficits

- LDOnline.org, http://www.ldonline.org
- Learning Disabilities Association of America, www.ldaamerica.org
- http://www.tsbvi.edu/Outreach/seehear/spring00/centralauditory.htm
- Discussion Group:
    - http://groups.yahoo.com/group/AuditoryProcessing — This list welcomes questions, comments, suggestions, insights, and concerns about APD and related matters.

Cerebral Palsy

- United Cerebral Palsy, www.ucp.org
- Discussion Group:
    - http://groups.yahoo.com/group/OurFrontPorch — for people with cerebral palsy and their families

Cleft Lip and Palate

(see Craniofacial Anomalies)

Craniofacial Anomalies

- AboutFace, www.aboutfaceusa.org
- American Cleft Palate-Craniofacial Association (ACPA), www.acpa-cpf.org
- RSF-EARTHSPEAK, www.rsf-earthspeak.org
- The Cleft Palate Foundation, www.cleftline.org
- Discussion Group:
    - http://groups.yahoo.com/group/cleftnotes— for families and individuals dealing with issues surrounding cleft lip and/or palate

Deaf

(see Hearing Impairments)

Dementia

(see Alzheimer's or Memory)

Developmental Disabilities and Delays

The Arc of the United States, www.thearc.org

- http://edchapman.tripod.com/ParentLinks.html — This site offers useful information such as developmental milestones, acronyms, links, and mailing lists for parents on speech delays, developmental delays, and special education.

- The Institute for the Achievement of Human Potential, www.iahp.org

- Discussion Groups

  - http://groups.yahoo.com/group/BirthtoThreeSupport — This group welcomes parents of children with any disability or at risk for a disability and professionals who work with these families.

  - http://groups.yahoo.com/group/childdevdelays/— This group offers support to parents of a child (or children) with developmental delays (speech and language, motor, cognitive, sensory, emotional and social, etc.).

  - http://groups.yahoo.com/group/Latetalkers — This group was formed to facilitate the discussion of developmental speech delays caused by apraxia (dyspraxia), phonological disorders, autism spectrum disorders, learning disabilities, or other causes.

Down Syndrome

- National Down Syndrome Society, www.ndss.org

- Discussion Group

  - **DOWN-SYN.** To subscribe to this list for Down Syndrome, send e-mail to listserv@listserv.nodak.edu with the message: subscribe down-syn firstname lastname. Send messages to all subscribers to down-syn@listserv.nodak.edu.

Dysarthria

(see Resources for Aphasia and Stroke)

Dyslexia

(see Resources for Learning Disabilities)

Epilepsy

- Epilepsy Foundation, www.epilepsyfoundation.org
- American Epilepsy Society, www.aesnet.org

English Language Learners (ELL)

- Center for Adult English Language Acquisition (CAELA) www.cal.org/caela/
- National Association for Bilingual Education, www.nabe.org
- National Council for Teachers of English, www.ncte.org
- Office of English Language Enhancement, www.ed.gov/about/offices/list/oela/index.html
- Teaching Diverse Learners (TDL), www.alliance.brown.edu/tdl/

English as a Second Language (ESL)

(see English Language Learners)

Executive Function Disorders

(see Brain Injury)

Fluency

(see Stuttering)

Head Injury

(see Brain Injury)

Hearing Impairment

- Hearing Loss Association of America, www.shhh.org

- National Deaf Education Center at Gallaudet University, http://clerccenter.gallaudet.edu/InfoToGo

- The Deaf Resource Library, http://www.deaflibrary.org

- Deafness/Hard of Hearing, presented by About.com, http://deafness.miningco.com/health/disabilities/deafness/msubdict.htm.

- Discussion Groups:

  - http://groups.yahoo.com/group/Listen-Up — for parents of deaf/hard of hearing children.

  - DEAF-L. A list for the discussion of questions, topics, and concerns related to deafness. To subscribe, send e-mail to listserv@siu.edu with the message: subscribe deaf-l firstname lastname. To communicate to the entire list, send the message to deaf-l@siu.edu.

Huntington's Disease

- Huntington's Disease Society of America, www.hdsa.org

- International Huntington Association, www.huntington-assoc.com

- Caring for People With Huntington's Disease, www.kumc.edu/hospital/huntingtons

Learning Disabilities

- Council for Learning Disabilities, www.cldinternational.org

- Dyslexia Research Institute (DRI), www.dyslexia-add.org

- Learning Disabilities Association of America, www.ldanatl.org

- LD Online, www.ldonline.org

- LD Resources at www.ldresources.com

- Literacy Connections, www.literacyconnections.com

- National Dissemination Center for Children With Disabilities (NICHCY), www.nichcy.org

- NLD on the Web, www.nldontheweb.org

- Roads to Learning, www.ala.org/olos/outreachresource/roadtolearning/roadslearning.htm

- Schwab Learning, www.schwablearning.org

- Discussion Group
  - http://groups.yahoo.com/group/DyslexiaSupport/— This list is for the discussion of dyslexia. It is a place to share ideas and exchange ways of helping, but not limited to, school aged children. Hopefully, this can be a place where professionals who work with dyslexia can provide tips and dyslexic adults and parents with dyslexic children can come for support.

Low Vision

(see Visual Impairments)

Memory

(see Alzheimer's and Brain Injury)

Multiple Sclerosis (MS)

- Destination Cure, www.destinationcure.com
- Multiple Sclerosis Association of America, www.msaa.com
- National MS Society, www.nationalmssociety.org

Parkinson Disease

- Parkinson's Disease Foundation, www.pdf.org
- Parkinson's Disease Society, www.parkinsons.org.uk (England)

Pervasive Developmental Disorder (PDD)

(see Autistic Spectrum Disorders)

Slurred Speech

(see Dysarthria)

Stroke

(see also Aphasia, Apraxia, Memory)

- American Heart Association, www.americanheart.org

- Hope for Stroke, www.hope4stroke.com

- Montgomery County Stroke Association, www.mcstroke.org

- National Stroke Association, www.stroke.org

- Heart and Stroke Foundation of Canada, http://ww2.heartandstroke.ca

- Discussion Groups

  - STROKE-L. To subscribe to this stroke discussion list, send e-mail to listserv@lsv.uky.edu with the message: subscribe stroke-l firstname lastname. To contribute to the list, send a message to stroke-l@lsv.uky.edu.

Stuttering

- The Stuttering Home Page by Judith Kuster, www.mnsu.edu/comdis/kuster/stutter.html

- The Stuttering Foundation of America, www.stutteringhelp.org

- National Stuttering Association, www.nsastutter.org

- Friends, The National Association of Young People Who Stutter, www.friendswhostutter.org

- Specialty Board on Fluency Disorders, www.stutteringspecialists.org

- Istutter, www.latrobe.edu.au/istutter

- The Onset and Development of stuttering video by Valerie LaPorte and Cindy Spillers, www.d.umn.edu/~cspiller/stutteringpage/onset.htm — There are video clips of seven danger signs of stuttering from the Stuttering Foundation of America's film "Prevention of Stuttering: Identifying the Danger Signs."

- Discussion Groups:

  - http://groups.yahoo.com/group/stutteringchat — for people who stutter and their friends, family, and clinicians.

  - PARENTS-W@EGROUPS.COM. A list for parents concerned about stuttering behaviors in children. Professionals, students, and others interested are also welcome to join. Subscribe at the following Web site: http://www.egroups.com/group/Parents-W.

- STUTT-L. To subscribe to this discussion list on stuttering research and clinical practice, send e-mail to listserv@listserv. temple.edu with the message: subscribe stutt-l firstname lastname. To contribute to the list, send message to stutt-l@vm.temple.edu.

- STUTT-X. To subscribe to this stuttering-communication disorders list, send e-mail to listserv@asu.edu with the message: subscribe stutt-x firstname lastname. To contribute to the list send message to stutt-x@asuvm.inre.asu.edu.

Traumatic Brain Injury

(see Brain Injury)

Unintelligible Speech

(see Accent Reduction, Apraxia, or Aphasia)

Visual Impairments

- National Association for Visually Handicapped (NAVH), www.navh.org
- American Foundation for the Blind, www.afb.org
- International Society for Low Vision Research and Rehabilitation's Vision Connection, www.visionconnection.org/VisionConnection/default.htm
- Lighthouse International, www.lighthouse.org
- Visions Matters, www.visionmatters.net

Voice

- VoiceDisorders.com, www.voiceproblem.org
- The Voice Foundation, www.voicefoundation.org

Sites With Information About Products To Promote Independent Living

- Abledata, www.abledata.com

- Alimed, www.alimed.com

- EnableMart, www.enablemart.com

- Family Village — Accessibility Shopping Mall, http://www.familyvillage.wisc.edu/mall.htm

- Freedom Living Devices, www.freedomlivingdevices.com

- Gold Violin, www.goldviolin.com

- Independent Living Aids, www.independentliving.com

- Interactive Therapeutics, www.interactivetherapy.com

- MAXI Aids, www.maxiaids.com

Sites Offering Assistive Technology Training and Information

AAC Connecting Young Kids (YAACK)
http://aac.unl.edu/yaack

- This Web site was developed by Ruth Ballinger and provides a good overview of augmentative and alternative communication (AAC).

- It has three main sections: Getting Started, Choosing a System, and Teaching Tips.

Ace Centre
http://ace-centre.hostinguk.com

- Provides an instructional handbook on PowerPoint Talking Books in PDF form.

Alliance for Technology Access (ATA)
www.ataccess.org/resources/atabook/default.html

- ATA produces the book *Computer and Web Resources for People with Disabilities: A Guide to Exploring Today's Assistive Technology*.

- The site also has an AT Mini-Assessment that can be downloaded and it includes a publication titled Assistive Technology in K-12 Schools.

Alternatively Speaking
available at www.augcominc.com

- This is an international, consumer-written, and consumer-edited publication in the field of augmentative and alternative communication.

- AS highlights the consumer's perspective.

- Three issues per year at an individual subscriber rate of $35.00 in the US.

Assistive Technology Training On Line
available at http://atto.buffalo.edu

- The Assistive Technology Training Online Project (ATTO) provides information on AT applications that help students with disabilities learn in elementary classrooms.

- There are four helpful sections with a wealth of helpful information — AT Basics, Tutorials, At Decision Making, and Resources.

- There is also a section that contains an overview the laws on civil rights, special education, and assistive technology arranged chronologically.

AT / AAC enables
available at http://depts.washington.edu/enables/index.htm

- This ever-developing, Web-based video resource is regularly updated by Patricia Dowden, Ph.D., CCC-Sp, Assistant Clinical Professor.

- It offers a searchable video archive with sections on:

- Dispelling Myths in AAC and AT

- Profiles of People Using AT and AAC

- AAC Video Museum

Atomic Learning
available at www.atomiclearning.com

- Atomic Learning provides Web-based software training for more than 100 applications students and educators use everyday.

- There are more than 20,000 tutorial movies on more than 100 applications and free online tutorials.

- Lesson Accelerators teach essential software skills while using tutorial movies to demonstrate, step-by-step, how to create curriculum-based technology projects.

- An annual subscription is $79.99.

Augmentative Communication News
available at www.augcominc.com

- Augmentative Communication News (ACN) is a quarterly publication written by Sarah Blackstone. This 8-page to 16-page news report features a range of "hot" topics in the area of AAC.

- An Individual subscriber rate is $50.00

Barkley AAC Center
available at http://aac.unl.edu/

- Provides AAC messaging and vocabulary

- Lists AAC Medicare resources

- Presents a wide variety of PowerPoint presentations on a variety of AAC topics.

Center for Applied Special Technology (CAST)
available at www.cast.org

- This site provides information on universal design and links in the areas of organizations, shareware, articles, vendors, publications, and Web authoring information.

Center for Disabilities (CSUN)
available at www.csun.edu/cod/conf/index.htm

- This site contains proceedings for all years of the Conference on Technology and Disabilities as well as many excellent papers on a variety of assistive technology applications and topics.

Closing the Gap
available at www.closingthegap.com

- Closing the Gap offers a variety of forums with useful information about AT, a place to request a free copy of their newsletter and excellent online directory of assistive technology.

- Access to the directory, a subscription to the newsletter and past issues of the newsletter require membership.

ConnSENSE Bulletin
available at http://connsensebulletin.com

- This site provides practical resources on assistive technology through a number of articles, resources, position papers, and current event updates.

The Early Childhood Technology Integrated Educational System (EC-TIIS)
available at www.wiu.edu

- Free on-line workshops for using technology with young children.

Education Word
available at www.education-world.com

- Education World's goal is to make it easy for educators to integrate the Internet into the classroom.

- A special section is available for technology integration resources. On that page there are sections titled: Tech in the classroom, Featured Articles, Tech Tips, Tech Projects, Columnists Podium, and Tech Tools.

Georgia Project for Assistive Technology
available at www.gpat.org,

- This site offers a vast number of resources that are organized by topic. They include narrative documents, PowerPoint presentations, forms, on-line videos, and Web links.

- Over 100 video clips show children using assistive technology that was developed in a collaborative effort with Valdosta State University.

- GPAT provides many assistive technology resource charts that can be downloaded.

InPictures
available at http://inpics.net/

- In Pictures provides free online tutorials are based on pictures, not words.

- The tutorial format is based on results from a research study for the U.S. Department of Education regarding how to make it easier for people with learning disabilities to learn computer subjects.

- This site currently includes Web-based tutorials on Microsoft office applications, Open Office applications, Web layout, and Web graphics.

- New tutorials are now being developed on Office 2007, Photoshop, MySQL, PHP, and Perl.

Internet4Classrooms
available at www.internet4classrooms.com

- A collection of online tutorials.

TASC (*Technology Assistance for Special Consumers*)
available at http://tasc.ataccess.org

- The section for Assistive Tools offers an informative introduction to AT.

- TASC provides many links to vendors of assistive technology.

Linda Burkhart
available at www.lburkhart.com

- This site by Linda Burkhart focuses on Technology Integration in Education with many excellent examples and suggestions.

- There are three main sections — AT in Elementary Schools, AT in Middle Schools and Special Needs.

National Assistive Technology Research Institute (NATRI)
available at http://natri.uky.edu

- NATRI offers a listing of resources for Assistive Technology.

- They link to external sites devoted to AT resources, information databases, AT vendors, and AT device locator systems.

- There are a few videos of selected resources.

National Assistive Technology in Education Network (NATE)
available at http://natenetwork.buffalo.edu

- NATE's mission is to help service providers develop their capacity to work collaboratively to implement assistive technology services that are legal, ethical, cost effective and efficient.

- It includes a variety of data collection forms, monographs to guide professionals who use assistive technology, professional support, tips for technology use, and many helpful technology resources.

Neighborhood Legal Services
available at http://www.nls.org/booklets.htm

- This company has written a series of booklets on legal and funding issues related to assistive technology.

- A single copy of each of them is available at no cost.

OATSoft
available at www.oatsoft.org

- OatSoft is dedicated to improving Assistive Technology and computer accessibility through the power of Open Source development techniques.

- There are useful guides for using assistive technology in education.

- It lists open source projects to help with tasks such as text input, communication, viewing the screen, accessing the Web and using the mouse.

- There is a section devoted to the development of assistive technology software.

Promoting Augmentative Communication Together (PACT)
available at http://groups.yahoo.com/group/pact/

- PACT is a community listserv for anyone interested in the field of augmentative and alternative communication (AAC).

- This listserv extends to people who use or need AAC, their families, and the various professionals who provide AAC services.

Quality Indicators of Assistive Technology (QIAT) Consortium
available at www.qiat.org

- This Web site contains a collection of many useful documents and tools related to assistive technology.

- It provides the opportunity to join the QIAT electronic mailing list where teachers, therapists, and family members routinely discuss assistive technology issues.

State AT Programs
available at www.resna.org/taproject/at/statecontacts.html

- The Technical Assistance Project is funded to assist people needing AT.

- This project also provides technical assistance in the areas related to universal design, state procurement actions, and funding of AT.

The TAM (Technology and Media) Division of the Council for Exceptional Children
available at www.tamcec.org

- TAM offers a variety of information about assistive technology and special education instructional technology.

TechLearning
available at www.techlearning.com

- This site is the online version of *Technology & Learning* magazine.

- A section called Educators' Outlook includes content for teachers, librarians, and media coordinators who want to use the Web in the classroom.

- Searchable information includes a database of sites, a directory of funding opportunities that lists grants available for teachers, and information for particular subject areas.

Technology: LD in Depth
available at www.LDOnLine.org

- Site includes Tech Talk, Technology Reviews, Classroom Applications, Tech Guide to Products, Technology Resources, and Integrating Technology.

- Tech Talk and articles can be downloaded.

Tuning in AT
available at http://tuninginat.blogspot.com

- Tuning In AT is a podcast for Adaptive Technologists to get the latest information on technology that can help students with disabilities.

Rehabilitation Engineering and Assistive Technology Society of North America (RESNA)
available at www. resna.org

- RESNA is an interdisciplinary association for the advancement of rehabilitation and assistive technologies (AT).

- Its listserv tends to be technical and encompasses all assistive technologies. It is an excellent place to obtain specific technical information on AAC.

- Information on how to subscribe to RESNA's listserv and to access its archives is at www.resna.org/sigs/sig11/resnalst.htm.

UW Augcomm
available at http://depts.washington.edu/augcomm/index.htm

- Describes a Continuum of Communication Independence that is helpful for intervention.

- Provides strategies for selecting AAC vocabularies.

- Reviews AAC features to consider during the selection process.

- Provides video clips, images, and stories about individuals using AT and AAC while participating in all aspects of life.

Wisconsin Assistive Technology Initiative- Resource Guide for Teachers and Administrators About Assistive Technology
available at www.wati.org

- WATI provides a 24-page downloadable PDF document that provides an excellent, easily understood overview of assistive technology. This booklet may be reproduced and is an excellent tool for training.

- Free forms are provided to help the user with the assessment process. It is referred to as the WATI Assistive Technology Consideration Guide.

- WATI also has a transition packet that can be downloaded. It contains a series of forms to guide the assembly of information necessary to support an AT user as he or she transitions to adult services. It includes assessment tools and planning sheets.

Valdosta State University in cooperation with the Georgia Project for AT
http://coefaculty.valdosta.edu/spe/ATRB/index.html

- This site offers excellent training modules including videos about a wide range of assistive technology devices and services.

Sites Grouped by Profession

These are very helpful sites to obtain resources for your profession or to research potential referral sources. Many of the sites offer listservs, blogs and e-newsletters.

Administrators/Directors

- American College of Healthcare Executives, www.ache.org/aboutache.cfm
- American Health Care Association, http://ahca.org
- American Association Healthcare Administrative Management, www.aaham.org
- American Association of School Administrators, www.aasa.org
- Association for Community Organization & Social Administration (ACOSA), www.acosa.org
- CITED Learn Center (Center for Implementing Technology in Education), www.cited.org
- Education & Disability Information Resources, www.hamptonu.edu/bsrc/CMSE/dinfo.html
- National Association for the Education of Young Children - www.naeyc.org
- National Association of Elementary School Principals, www.naesp.org
- National Association for Secondary School Principals, www.prinicpals.org
- National Association of State Directors of Special Education, Inc. (NASDSE), www.nasdse.org
- National Council on Disability, www.ncd.gov
- National Council on Rehabilitation Education, www.rehabeducators.org
- National Middle School Association, www.nmsa.org
- National Rehabilitation Information Center, www.naric.com
- US Department of Education, www.ed.gov

Audiologists

- Academy of Rehabilitative Audiology, www.audrehab.org
- American Academy of Audiology, www.audiology.com
- American Speech- Language and Hearing Association, www.asha.org

- Audiology Information Network, www.audiologyinfo.com
- Canadian Association of Speech-Language Pathologists and Audiologists, www.caslpa.ca

Case Managers

- American Case Management Association, www.acmaweb.org
- Case Management Resource Guide, www.cmrg.com
- National Association for Professional Geriatric Case Managers, www.caremanager.org

Gerontologists

- The Gerontological Society of America, www.geron.org

Graduate Students

- Gradschools.com, www.gradschools.com
- Graduate Guide, www.graduateguide.com

Learning Disability Specialists

- Council for Learning Disabilities (CLD), www.cldinternational.org
- International Dyslexia Association, www.interdys.org
- Internet Special Education Resources (ISER), www.iser.com
- Learning Disabilities Association of America, www.ldaamerica.org
- National Association of Special Education Teachers, www.naset.org
- Professionals in Learning Disabilities, www.pldonline.org
- SchwabLearning.org, www.schwablearning.org
- Special Education Resources on the Internet (SERI), www.seriweb.com

Media Specialists

(See Technology Coordinators)

Neurologists

- American Medical Association, www.ama-assn.org

- Canadian Congress of Neurological Sciences, www.ccns.org

Neuropsychologists

- American Academy of Clinical Neuropsychology, www.theaacn.org
- American Board of Clinical Neuropsychology, www.theabcn.org
- American Psychological Association- Clinical Neuropsychology, www.div40.org
- International Neuropsychological Society, www.the-ins.org
- Neuropsychology Central, www.neuropsychologycentral.com

Occupational Therapists

- American Occupational Therapy Association, www.aota.org
- Canadian Association of Occupational Therapists, www.caot.ca
- World Federation of Occupational Therapists, www.wfot.org.au

Pediatricians

- American Academy of Pediatrics (AAP), www.aap.org

Physiatrists

- American Academy of Physical Medicine and Rehabilitation, www.aapmr.org
- Canadian Association of Physical Medicine and Rehabilitation, http://capmr.medical.org

Recreational Therapists

- American Therapeutic Recreation Association, www.atra-tr.org
- National Coalition of Creative Art Therapies, www.nccata.com
- Society for Arts in HealthCare, http://thesah.org

Social Workers/Counselors

- American Mental Health Counselors Association, www.amhca.org
- Human Service Information Technology Applications, www.husita.org
- International Federation of Social Workers, www.ifsw.org

- National Network for Social Work Managers, www.socialworkmanager.org
- National Association of Social Workers, www.socialworkers.org
- Social Work Access Network (SWAN), http://cosw.sc.edu/swan

Special Education Teachers

(see Learning Disability Specialists and Teachers)

Speech-Language Pathologists

- American Association of Private Practice in Speech Pathology and Audiology (AAPPSPA), www.aappspa.org
- American Speech-Language-Hearing Association, www.asha.org
- Council of Academic Programs in Communication Sciences and Disorders (CAPCSD), www.capcsd.org
- Canadian Association of Speech-Language Pathologists and Audiologists, www.caslpa.ca
- Net Connections for Communication Disorders and Sciences, www.mnsu.edu/comdis/kuster2/welcome.html
- University Programs in Speech-Language Pathology and Audiology by Scott Bradley, http://facstaff.uww.edu/bradleys/cdprograms.html.
- Discussion Groups- Most Special Interest Groups (SIGs) offer online discussion groups. ASHA members who belong to the groups may find out more information at www.asha.org.

Teachers

- American Federation of Teachers, www.aft.org
- CITED Action Center (Center for Implementing Technology in Education), www.cited.org
- Computer Using Educators, www.cue.org
- Internet 4 Classrooms, www.internet4classrooms.com
- National Council of the Teachers of English, www.ncte.org
- National Education Association, www.nea.org
- School World, www.schoolworld.com
- The Access Center, www.k8accesscenter.org

Technology Coordinator/Media Specialist

- CITED Learn Center (Center for Implementing Technology in Education), www.cited.org
- Technology Coordinators Handbook, www.schools.pinellas.k12.fl.us/tchandbk/default.htm
- Discussion Group
  - Technology Coordinator's Listserv — To sign up, e-mail macjordomo@alisal.org and write "subscribe techcoord" in the body.

Tutors

- National Tutoring Association, www.ntatutor.org

University Professors

- American Association of University Professors, www.aaup.org

Vendors/Software Developers

- The Alliance for Technology Access, www.ataccess.org
- Assistive Technology Industry Association, www.atia.org

Vocational Counselors

- DisabilityInfo.gov, www.disabilityinfo.gov
- International Association of Rehabilitation Professionals (IARP), www.rehabpro.org
- The Vocational Evaluation and Career Assessment Professionals (VECAP), www.vecap.org
- Vocational Rehabilitation Association, (VRA), (England) http://www.vocationalrehabilitationassociation.org.uk
- Voceval.com, www.voceval.com

Index of Vendors

Index of Products

Glossary of Technology, Education, and Rehabilitation Terms

Abbreviation Expansion

A feature of some software programs that allows the user to assign a series of letters, words, or sentences to one or more keystrokes

Accessibility Features

Product options that enable a user to adjust settings to accommodate his or her visual, mobility, hearing, language, or learning needs

Accessible Technology

Software and hardware that may assist with communication, cognition, mobility, vision, and hearing

Accommodations

Changes made to the environment (school, home, work) to enable people to function more independently

Acquired

Something that occurs after birth

Activities of Daily Living (ADL)

Routine activities that are performed day to day, such as getting dressed, preparing meals, doing household chores, working at a job, going to school, and using transportation

Adaptations

Specific accommodations, modifications, and supports to help people compensate for challenges and functional limitations

Advocacy

The representation of a person's best interests

Aids for Activities for Daily Living (ADL)

Self-help aids for use in activities such as eating, bathing, shopping, and home maintenance

Alerting Devices

An accommodation for people that emits visual or tactile signals

Alternative Input Device

A device such as an alternative keyboard, electronic pointing device, or touch screen that enables a person to control his or her computer in a way other than by a standard keyboard

Amplification

Increasing the loudness of sounds

Aneurysm

A balloon-like deformity in the wall of a blood vessel: The wall weakens as the balloon grows larger and may eventually burst, causing a hemorrhage

Anomia

The inability to recall the names of objects: People with this problem often can speak fluently, but have to use other words to describe familiar objects

Anti-virus software

Computer programs designed to detect the presence or occurrence of a computer virus. The software subsequently signals an alert and can be used to delete the virus

Aphasia

Total or partial loss of the ability to use or understand language; usually caused by stroke, brain disease, or injury

Aphasia, Fluent

Communication that is characterized by spontaneous use of language at normal speed that conveys little meaning: There is typically poor comprehension with fluent aphasia.

Aphasia, Non-fluent

Characterized by awkward articulation; limited vocabulary; hesitant, slow speech output; restricted use of grammatical forms; and a relative preservation of auditory comprehension

Aphasia, Receptive

Problems in understanding what others attempt to communicate

Aphonia

Complete loss of voice

Application software

Computer programs that are used to accomplish specific tasks not related to the computer itself: Examples are word processors, text readers, voice-recognition software, and spreadsheets.

Apraxia

The inability to execute a voluntary movement despite being able to demonstrate normal muscle function

Articulation Disorder

An inability to correctly produce speech sounds (phonemes) because of imprecise placement, timing, pressure, speed, or flow of movement of the lips, tongue, or throat

Assessment

A process by which a team of highly trained professionals observes and evaluates an individual to determine level of performance and needs

Assistive Devices

Technical tools and devices such as alphabet boards, text telephones, or text-to-speech conversion software used to aid individuals who have communication disorders perform actions, tasks, and activities

Assistive Listening Devices (ALDs)

Supplementary electronic devices to help people hear more directly

Assistive Technology (AT)

Any product, device, or equipment that is used to maintain, increase, or improve the functional capabilities of individuals with disabilities

Attention Deficit Hyperactivity Disorder (ADHD)

Hyperactivity and attentional difficulties in children who do not show other characteristics of learning disabilities

Attention/Concentration, Distractibility

A person's inability to sustain attention because of competing internal or external stimuli

Attention, Divided

An attentional task, requiring to two or more inputs or activities at the same time

Attention/Concentration, Length

The length of time a person is able to focus on a given task. Complexity of task and fatigue will affect length of attention (attention span)

Audiologist

A health care professional who is trained to evaluate hearing loss and related disorders

Auditory Feedback

A sound that is produced in response to a user's action: It may be a short sound, spoken words or spoken label.

Auditory Perception

The ability to identify, to interpret, and to attach meaning to sound

Automatic Speech

Words said without much thinking on the part of the speaker: These may include songs, numbers, and social communication. It can also be items previously learned through memorization.

Augmentative and Alternative Communication (AAC)

An area of clinical practice that helps people compensate for significant speech limitations by supplementing or establishing a verbal communication system

Augmentative and assistive communication devices

Tools used by a person who is unable to express himself verbally: The user types words or phrases or selects one or more pictures that can generate a message said aloud by the device.

Authoring Software Program

Software that provides a method or style of delivery, but provides either no content or the ability to customize the content/stimuli items used in the program

Autism

A brain disorder that begins in early childhood; affects communication, social interaction, and creative or imaginative play

Aural Rehabilitation

Techniques used with people who are hearing impaired to improve their ability to speak and communicate

Awareness Deficit

The client's inability to recognize the problems caused by impaired brain function

Brain Injury

Damage to the brain that results in impairments in one or more functions, including arousal, attention, language, memory, reasoning, abstract thinking, judgment, problem solving, sensory abilities, perceptual abilities, motor abilities, psychosocial behavior, information processing, and speech: The damage may be caused by external physical force, insufficient blood supply, toxic substances, malignancy, disease-producing organisms, congenital disorders, birth trauma, or degenerative processes.

Brain Plasticity

The ability of intact brain cells to take over functions of damaged cells

Browsers

Software programs that interpret the code used to create Web sites and present it in an intelligible format

Captioning

The conversion of audio into text that can be read on a screen

Case Management

The coordination and delivery of medical, rehabilitation, and support programs to a person

Categorization

A grouping of objects based on similar attributes

Chat Room

A virtual room on the Internet where people communicate with each other almost immediately: They normally chat by typing messages to each other, but they may also use new technology that allows them to use their voices.

Chronic Care

Long-term care for people who require medical care, a maintenance program to prevent deterioration of skills, and recreational and social opportunities in a structured environment

Central Auditory Processing Disorder (CAPD)

A CAPD is a receptive language disorder. It refers to difficulties in the decoding and storing of auditory information — usually incoming verbal messages

Cerebral Palsy (CP)

A motor disorder produced by damage to the brain early in life

Circumlocution

The use of other words to describe a specific word or idea that cannot be remembered

Client

In this guide, a person who engages the professional advice or services of another: Clients can also be consumers, patients, and students.

Clinician

In this guide, refers to a wide range of professionals who may be involved in helping the clients who have communication and cognitive impairments

Cloze Techniques

A method of asking a client to restore the omitted portion of an oral or written message for its remaining context

Cognition

Thinking skills that include perception, memory, awareness, reasoning, judgment, intellect, and imagination

Cognitive Deficits

Difficulty attending to and appropriately responding to information

Cognitive Rehabilitation

Therapy programs that aid people in the management of specific problems in perception, memory, thinking, and problem solving: Skills are practiced and strategies are taught to help improve function and/or compensate for remaining deficits. The interventions are based on an assessment and understanding of the person's brain-behavior deficits.

Communication Disorder

An impairment in the ability to receive and/or process a symbol system, represent concepts or symbol systems, and/or transmit and use symbol systems:

The impairment may be observed in disorders of hearing, language, and/or speech processes.

Community Resources

Public or private agencies, schools, or programs offering services, usually funded by governmental bodies, community drives, donations, and fees

Community Skills

Abilities that are needed to function independently in the community: They may include telephone skills, money management, pedestrian skills, using public transportation, meal planning, and cooking.

Comprehension

Understanding of spoken, written, or gestural communication

Concentration

Maintaining attention on a task over a period of time; remaining attentive and being not easily diverted

Concrete Thinking

A style of thinking in which the individual sees each situation as unique and is unable to generalize from the similarities between situations: Language and perceptions are interpreted literally.

Concussion

The common result of a blow to the head or sudden deceleration usually causing an altered mental state, either temporary or prolonged: Physiologic and/or anatomic disruption of connections between some nerve cells in the brain may occur.

Confabulation

Verbalizations about people, places, and events with no basis in reality

Congenital Disability

A disability that has existed since birth, but is not necessarily hereditary

Cue

A signal or direction used to assist a person in performing an activity

Cursor

The pointer or marker that indicates where you are on the computer screen

Day Care

A service provided during ordinary working hours for the person who requires supervision: It can include assistance with medication, meal preparation, dressing, or moving about. The family or other caregiver returns the person to their residence and assumes responsibility for care during the evenings and at night.

Deaf

A profound degree of hearing loss that prevents understanding of speech received through the ear: "Hearing impaired" is the generic term preferred by some individuals to refer to any degree of hearing loss, from mild to profound. It includes both hard of hearing and deaf. "Hard of hearing" refers to a mild to moderate hearing loss that may or may not be corrected with amplification.

Developmental Disability

Any mental and/or physical disability that has an onset before age twenty-two and may continue indefinitely: It can limit major life activities. The term includes individuals with mental retardation, cerebral palsy, autism, epilepsy (and other seizure disorders), sensory impairments, congenital disabilities, traumatic accidents, or conditions caused by disease.

Disability

An impairment that substantially affects one or more major life activities

Discrimination, Auditory

The ability to differentiate and recognize sounds: This involves distinguishing between words, noises, and sounds that might be similar.

Discrimination, Visual

Involves the differentiation of items using sight

Disinhibition

The inability to suppress (inhibit) impulsive behavior and emotions

Disorientation

Not knowing where you are, who you are, or the current date

Divergent Thinking

A thought process during which a person explores ideas and concepts that fan out from an initial concept

Download

The process of transfer files from the Internet or a computer to another

Down's Syndrome

A form of mental retardation and congenital anomaly caused by improper chromosomal division during fetal development

Dysphagia

A swallowing disorder characterized by difficulty in oral preparation for the swallow or in moving material from the mouth to the stomach: This also includes problems in positioning food in the mouth.

Dysgraphia

A neurological disorder characterized by writing disabilities

Dysarthria

A group of speech disorders caused by disturbances in the strength or coordination of the muscles of the speech mechanism as a result of damage to the brain or nerves

Dysfluency

A disruption in the smooth flow or expression of speech

Dyslexia

A learning disability characterized by reading difficulties: Some individuals may also have difficulty writing, spelling, or working with numbers.

Dysphonia

An impairment of the voice or speaking ability

Dyspraxia of Speech

The partial loss of the ability to consistently pronounce words in individuals with normal muscle tone and speech muscle coordination

Early Intervention Services

A program of activities and services for children from birth through age two that emphasizes cognitive, communication, motor, and social skills

Educational Consultant

An individual who may be familiar with school curriculum and requirements at various grade levels: They may or may not have a background in learning disabilities and may conduct educational evaluations.

Electronic Pointing Device

A tool that controls the cursor placement on the screen: When used with an on-screen keyboard, it can be used to enter text or data.

Evidence-Based Research

A process that that gathers evidence to answer questions and bring new knowledge to a field so that effective practice can be determined and implemented

Executive Functions

Planning, prioritizing, sequencing, self-monitoring, self-correcting, inhibiting, initiating, controlling, or altering behavior

Extended Skilled Care Facility

A residential facility for the patient who requires 24-hour nursing care and rehabilitation therapy: Therapies can include physical therapy, occupational therapy, or speech therapy on a less intensive basis than as an inpatient in a comprehensive rehabilitation center. An extended care facility can be a short-term alternative (a few months) prior to placement at home (with outpatient therapy) or in a nursing home.

Feedback

The method used to respond to a person's actions: Computer feedback may be auditory, visual, or multi-sensory.

Filter keys

An accessibility option in Windows that adjusts the keyboard response so that unwanted repeated strokes that may be caused by a tremor are ignored

Firewalls

A system designed to prevent unauthorized access to a private network: Firewalls can be implemented in both hardware and software

Frontal Lobe

The front part of the brain involved in planning, organizing, problem solving, selective attention, personality, and a variety of higher cognitive functions

Frustration Tolerance

The ability to persist in completing a task despite apparent difficulty: Individuals with a poor frustration tolerance will often refuse to complete tasks that are the least bit difficult.

Functional Ability

The capacity to perform an act that results in a practical end result

Graphic Organizers

Software programs that provide visual guides for brainstorming and organizing ideas

Hardware

The computer equipment used to run software programs: It consists of the items you can touch, such as the computer case and the peripherals (e.g., monitor, keyboard, mouse) that are attached to the computer.

Head Injury

Refers to an injury of the head and/or brain, including lacerations and contusions of the head, scalp, and/or forehead (Also refer to *brain injury.*)

Hearing Impaired

A generic term preferred by some individuals to refer to any degree of hearing loss, from mild to profound: It includes both hard of hearing and deaf

Hematoma

The collection of blood in tissues or space following the rupture of a blood vessel

Hemianopsia

A visual field cut: This is not the right or left eye, but the right or left half of vision in each eye.

Hemiparesis

A weakness of one side of the body

Hemiplegia

Paralysis of one side of the body because of injury to neurons carrying signals to muscles from the motor areas of the brain

Hemorrhage

Bleeding that occurs following damage to blood vessels: Bleeding may occur within the brain when blood vessels in the brain are damaged.

High Level Cognitive Processes

Refers to judgment, comprehension of problems, deductive and inductive reasoning, problem-solving, and planning

High Tech

Primarily refers to computerized or sophisticated electronic devices

Hypertext

Any text in web documents that contain "links" to other documents: Highlighted words or phrases in the document can be chosen by a reader to retrieve and display other documents.

Icon

A small picture representing something: Clicking an icon on a computer screen frequently activates a function of the computer such as opening a page.

IEP- Individualized Education Plan

A program customized for a learner with goals and required assistance

Initiative

A person's ability to begin a series of behaviors directed toward a goal

Input

Information a computer user provides to a computer: This may be typing text or talking into a microphone.

Instructional software

Computer programs that allow users to learn new content, practice using content already learned, and/or be evaluated on how much they know

Interactive

In software, a program feature that allows the user to make choices and cause actions

Interdisciplinary Approach

A method of diagnosis, evaluation, and individual program planning in which two or more specialists, such as medical doctors, teachers, speech pathologists, social workers, or occupational therapists, participate as a team: They contribute their skills, competencies, insights, and perspectives to focus on identifying the developmental needs of the person with a disability and on devising ways to meet those needs.

Interface

The connection between a computer and the person trying to use it: It can also be the connections required between computer systems so that communication and exchanges of data can take place.

ISP (Internet Service Provider)

An entity that provides commercial access to the Internet

Jargon

Spoken language that has normal rate and rhythm, but is full of nonsense words

JPEG (Joint Photographic Experts Group)

Pronounced *jay-peg*. A widely used standard for still, color images: The term is now used to label computer files containing pictures conforming to the standard.

Judgment

Process of forming an opinion, based upon an evaluation of the situation at hand in comparison with personal values, preferences, and insights regarding expected consequences

Key Guards

Covers with holes for each key to help people avoid selected unwanted keys

Language Disorders

Any of a number of problems with verbal communication and the ability to use or understand a symbol system for communication

Learning Disabilities

Childhood disorders characterized by difficulty with certain skills such as reading or writing in individuals with normal intelligence

Least Restrictive Environment

An environment (work, school, home) that provides a person with disabilities the chance to work and learn to the best of his or her ability: It also provides as much interaction as possible with people who do not have disabilities.

Level of Representation

The concreteness with which a target is symbolized: Some people recognize a target with photos, but not when they read the word or see a line drawing

Listservs

Provide e-mail messages for subscribers from other subscribers or exclusively from the owner of the listserv: Many listservs enable people to read archives (old messages) and to receive posting over a period of time in a form called a "digest."

Local Area Network (LAN)

The linkage of computers and/or peripherals such as Internet access and printers: The LAN is confined to a limited area that may consist of a room, building, or campus. This allows users to communicate and share information.

Log on

To connect to a computer or network, usually through the entry of an acceptable user ID and password

Low Tech

Typically refers to low cost and non-electronic devices

Mainstreaming

Integrating people with disabilities into the "least restrictive" setting: This often implies placement in a regular school classroom with special educational assistance, where necessary.

Management System

In software, the part of the program that tracks performance and summarizes scores

Menu

In software, it is the set up options available that allows the user to change settings, print, and exit the program

Memory

The process of organizing and storing representations of events and recalling these representations to consciousness at a later time

Memory, Auditory-Visual

Auditory memory is the ability to recall a series of numbers, lists of words, sentences, or paragraphs presented orally. Visual memory requires input of information through visual-perceptual channels. It refers to the ability to recall text, geometric figures, maps, and photographs.

Menu

A list of options or choices shown on the computer screen for user selection

Misarticulation

Inaccurately produced speech sound (phoneme) or sounds

Motor Speech Disorders

Group of disorders caused by the inability to accurately produce speech sounds (phonemes) because of muscle weakness or incoordination or difficulty performing voluntary muscle movements

Multimedia

The simultaneous use of sound, text, music, color, graphics, video, and/or animation

Multi-sensory

Any learning activity that includes the use of two or more sensory modalities simultaneously for the taking in or expression of information: It can involve auditory, visual, tactile-kinesthetic, and/or articulatory-motor components

Neologism

Nonsense or made-up word used when speaking: The person often does not realize that the word makes no sense.

Neglect

Paying little or no attention to a part of the body

Neural Stimulation

To activate or energize a nerve through an external source

Neurogenic Communication Disorder

The inability to exchange information with others because of hearing, speech, or language problems caused by impairment of the nervous system (brain or nerves)

Neurologist

A physician who specializes in disorders of the brain and nervous system

Neuroplasticity

The ability of the brain and/or certain parts of the nervous system to adapt to new conditions, such as an injury

Neuropsychologist

A psychologist who specializes in evaluating (by tests) brain/behavior relationships, planning training programs to help the survivor of brain injury return to normal functioning, and recommending alternative cognitive and behavioral strategies to minimize the effects of brain injury

Occipital Lobe

The region in the back of the brain that processes visual information Damage to this lobe can cause visual deficits

Occupational Therapy

Occupational therapy is the therapeutic use of self-care, work, and play activities to increase independent function, enhance development, and prevent disability. It may include the adaptation of a task or the environment to achieve maximum independence and to enhance the quality of life: The term "occupation," as used in occupational therapy, refers to any activity engaged in for evaluating, specifying, and treating problems interfering with functional performance.

On-Screen Keyboard

A keyboard appears on a computer monitor and can be accessed with a mouse or alternative pointing device

Optical Character Recognition (OCR)

Translates scanned text into a file that can be edited

Oral Apraxia

A neurological impairment in programming and executing speech and nonspeech movements of the mouth

Oral Motor

Has to do with the movement and placement of the oral structures such as the tongue, lips, palate, and teeth: Oral motor skills include the ability to lick your lips, stick out your tongue, and blow bubbles.

Output

The information a computer user receives from a computer, such as text on the monitor or voice output through speakers

Parietal Lobe

One of the two parietal lobes of the brain located behind the frontal lobe at the top of the brain: Damage to the right parietal lobe can cause visual-spatial deficits, awareness of deficits, and cognition. Damage to the left parietal lobe may disrupt a patient's ability to understand spoken and/or written language.

Perseveration

The inappropriate persistence of a response in a current task that may have been appropriate for a former task: Perseverations may be verbal or motoric.

Pervasive Developmental Disorders (PDD)

Disorders characterized by delays in several areas of development that may include socialization and communication

Phoneme

A family of speech sounds that are phonetically similar: Phonemes combine with each other to form words, phrases, and sentences.

Phonological Awareness

Involves the ability to notice, think about, or manipulate sound segments in words: It can include rhyming; syllable counting; detecting first, last, and middle sounds; and segmenting, adding, deleting, and substituting sounds in words.

Phonology

The study of speech sounds

Physiatrist

A physician who specializes in physical medicine and rehabilitation: Some physiatrists are experts in neurologic rehabilitation and are trained to diagnose and treat disabling conditions. The physiatrist examines the patient to assure that medical issues are addressed and provides appropriate medical information to the patient, family members, and members of the treatment team. The physiatrist follows the patient closely throughout treatment and oversees the patient's rehabilitation program.

Physical Therapist

The physical therapist evaluates components of movement, including muscle strength, muscle tone, posture, coordination, endurance, and general mobility. The physical therapist also evaluates the potential for functional movement, such as ability to move in bed, transfers, and walking. He or she then proceeds to establish an individualized treatment program to help the patient achieve functional independence.

Plateau

A temporary or permanent leveling off in the recovery process

Problem-Solving Skill

The ability to consider the probable factors that can influence the outcome of each of various solutions to a problem and to select the most advantageous solution

Prognosis

The prospect of recovery from a disease or injury, as indicated by the nature and symptoms of the case

Prosody

The melody of speech

Psychologist

A professional specializing in counseling, including adjustment to disability: Psychologists use tests to identify personality and cognitive functioning.

Quality of Life

A rating of what kind of existence a person experiences: In estimating the quality of life, the following items are usually considered: mobility and activities of daily life, living arrangements, social relationships, work and leisure activities, present satisfaction and future prospects.

Reading Disorders

Any of a group of problems characterized by difficulty using or understanding the symbol system for written language

Reasoning

The ability to take information, rules, and strategies learned about one situation and apply them appropriately to other situations

Receptive Language

Understanding words that are heard or read, even though hearing is fine

Rehabilitation

A comprehensive program to reduce and overcome deficits following injury or illness and to assists the individual in attaining the optimal level of mental and physical ability

Rehearsal

The process of repeating the same action or exercise several times in order to memorize it

Respite Care

A means of taking over the care of a patient temporarily to provide a period of relief for the primary caregiver

Scanners

A device that converts an image from a printed page to a computer file

Scanning

The active search of the environment for information: It usually refers to "visual scanning," which is a skill used in reading, driving, and many other daily activities.

Scanning is also a computer access method for switch users. Choices on the screen are highlighted one at a time and the user indicates a choice by activating an input device.

Screen Magnification

A computer program that enlarges the size of text and graphics shown on a monitor

Screen or Text Reader

Software that reads computer text and "speaks" it through voice output from the computer

Search Engines

Compares keywords typed in by the user to information provided by the search engine and presents them to the user

Seizure

An uncontrolled discharge of nerve cells that may spread to other cells nearby or throughout the entire brain: It usually lasts only few minutes.

Selective Attention

The ability to focus on the most important aspect of a situation without becoming distracted

Self-Advocacy

The awareness, motivation, and ability of an individual to communicate his or her own interests and exert control over his or her environment

Sequencing

Reading, listening, expressing thoughts, describing events, or performing a physical task in an orderly and meaningful manner

Social Worker

The social worker serves as a liaison between the professional team and other parties concerned with the patient, including the family, funding sources, friends, and representatives of past or future placements.

Speech

Spoken communication

Speech Disorder

Any defect or abnormality that prevents an individual from communicating by means of spoken words: Speech disorders may develop from developmental delays and disorders, nerve injury to the brain, muscular paralysis, structural defects, or intellectual impairment.

Speech-Language Pathologist

A health professional trained to evaluate and treat people who have voice, speech, language, cognitive, or swallowing disorders that affect their ability to communicate and think

Streaming Video

The sequence of "moving images" that are sent in compressed form over the Internet and displayed by the viewer as they arrive: Streaming media is streaming video with sound. With streaming video or streaming media, a Web user does not have to wait to download a large file before seeing the video or hearing the sound. Instead, the media is sent in a continuous stream and is played as it arrives.

Stroke

A stroke is also known as a cerebrovascular accident (CVA) or brain attack. It is caused by a lack of blood to the brain which results in the sudden loss of speech, language, or the ability to move a body part, and, if severe enough, death.

Stuttering

Frequent repetition of words or parts of words that disrupts the smooth flow of speech

Suite

A collection of software programs that are sold together and are supposed to work together efficiently and use similar commands

Support Group

A group established for families and/or persons with disabilities to discuss the problems they may have in coping with their life situation and to seek solutions to these problems

Surfing

Exploring locations and scanning the contents of Web sites on the Internet

Synthesized Speech

The speech of a computer, that is, the joining together of written letters, words, and numbers: A variety of voices are available that sound similar to human speech.

Sticky Keys

An accessibility option available on Windows that allows people with limited hand or fine motor control to use one finger to type multiple keys that are supposed to be pressed at the same time

Switches

Switches offer ways to provide input to a computer when a more direct access method, such as a keyboard or a mouse, is not possible. They come in a variety of sizes, shapes, placement options, and activation methods.

Tactile

Related to touch or the sense of touch

Talking Word Processor

A software program that uses speech synthesizers to provide auditory feedback of what is typed

Telegraphic Speech

Speech that sounds like a telegram: Only the main words of a sentence (nouns, verbs) are present. The small words (ifs, ands, buts,) are missing. This type of speech often gets the message across.

Text-Messaging

Typed messages are sent over phone lines

Text to Speech

The conversion of typed words to a spoken version, using a computer-generated voice

Toggle Keys

An accessibility feature in Windows that provides sounds cues when Caps Lock, Num Lock, or Shift keys are pressed

Touch Screen

A device that can be built-in or attached to a monitor; allows direct selection of the computer by touching the screen

Trackball

A type of alternative input device that uses a movable ball on top of a stationary base

Tracheostomy

Surgical opening into the trachea (windpipe) to help someone breathe who has an obstruction or swelling in the larynx (voice box) or upper throat or who has had the larynx surgically removed

Universal Design

A device or program is produced while taking into account the varying learning styles and needs of potential users — with and without disabilities

Version

The version number changes when a software developer makes major alterations to the software, such as adding new features.

Video Conferencing

With the use of a high-speed Internet connection and web cam, people can communicate over a long distance.

Vocal Cord Paralysis

The inability of one or both vocal folds (vocal cords) to move because of damage to the brain or nerves

Vocal Cords (Vocal Folds)

Folds of mucous membrane that extend from the larynx (voice box) wall: The folds are enclosed in elastic vocal ligament and muscle that control the tension and rate of vibration of the cords as air passes through them.

Vocational Rehabilitation Services

A range of services related to work, including training, counseling, job placement, and assistive technology

Voice

Sound produced by air passing out through the larynx and upper respiratory tract

Voice Disorders

A group of problems involving abnormal pitch, loudness, or quality of the sound produced by the larynx (voice box)

Voice/ Speech Recognition Software

A product that enables a user to enter text using his or her voice: Some software that uses voice recognition can also provide feedback regarding the accuracy of the speech/voice used.

Wi-Fi

A wireless technology that allows high-speed access to the network or Internet: A person with a Wi-Fi-enabled device, such as a computer, cell phone, or personal digital assistant (PDA) can connect to the Internet when in proximity of an access point often referred to as a "hotspot."

Wireless/Handheld Devices

Devices such as cell phones, Pocket PCs, Palm-powered devices, GPS receivers, and pagers that can be used to make and receive phone calls, text messages, and multimedia messages: These devices can keep track of schedules and address book information, play games and browse the Internet.

Word Completion Software

A type of program that enables the user to start to type a word and then presents choices of possible target words based on the letters typed

Word Prediction Software

A computer program that displays probable words as the user types

Word Processor

A computer program that allows a user to enter and revise text

Notes